AF734907

UP TO DATE ON MÉNIÈRE'S DISEASE

Edited by **Fayez Bahmad Jr**

Up to Date on Ménière's Disease
http://dx.doi.org/10.5772/62973
Edited by Fayez Bahmad Jr

Contributors

Ricardo Figueiredo, Andréia Azevedo, Norma Penido, Sankalp Gokhale, Shazia Mirza, Dinesh Sharma, Madalina Georgescu, Eduardo Amaro Bogaz, André Freitas Cavallini Da Silva, Davi Knoll Ribeiro, Gabriel Santos De Freitas, Fatih Oghan, Ibrahim Erdim, Bahadir Baykal, Ahmet Uluat, Onur Erdogan, Sinan Aksoy, Muhammet Fatih Topuz, Metin Celiker, Stavros Hatzopoulos, Andrea Ciorba, Piotr Henryk Skarzynski, Virginia Corazzi, Holger A. Rambold, Jess Tyrrell, Cassandra Phoenix, Sarah Bell, Aliciane Mota Cavalcante, Liane Sousa Teixeira, Alleluia Lima Losno Ledesma, Monique Barreto, Carlos Augusto C. P. Oliveira, Pauliana Lamounier, Fayez Bahmad

Published by InTech
Janeza Trdine 9, 51000 Rijeka, Croatia

© The Editor(s) and the Author(s) 2017
The moral rights of the editor(s) and the author(s) have been asserted.
All rights to the book as a whole are reserved by InTech. The book as a whole (compilation) cannot be reproduced, distributed or used for commercial or non-commercial purposes without InTech's written permission. Enquiries concerning the use of the book should be directed to InTech's rights and permissions department (permissions@intechopen.com).
Violations are liable to prosecution under the governing Copyright Law.

(cc) BY

Individual chapters of this publication are distributed under the terms of the Creative Commons Attribution 3.0 Unported License which permits commercial use, distribution and reproduction of the individual chapters, provided the original author(s) and source publication are appropriately acknowledged. More details and guidelines concerning content reuse and adaptation can be found at http://www.intechopen.com/copyright-policy.html.

Notice

Statements and opinions expressed in the chapters are these of the individual contributors and not necessarily those of the editors or publisher. No responsibility is accepted for the accuracy of information contained in the published chapters. The publisher assumes no responsibility for any damage or injury to persons or property arising out of the use of any materials, instructions, methods or ideas contained in the book.

Publishing Process Manager Romina Skomersic
Technical Editor SPi Global
Cover InTech Design team

First published October, 2017
Printed in Croatia
Legal deposit, Croatia: National and University Library in Zagreb

Additional hard copies can be obtained from orders@intechopen.com

Up to Date on Ménière's Disease, Edited by Fayez Bahmad Jr
p. cm.
Print ISBN 978-953-51-3419-0
Online ISBN 978-953-51-3420-6

We are IntechOpen, the first native scientific publisher of Open Access books

3,450+
Open access books available

110,000+
International authors and editors

115M+
Downloads

151
Countries delivered to

Our authors are among the
Top 1%
most cited scientists

12.2%
Contributors from top 500 universities

WEB OF SCIENCE™

Selection of our books indexed in the Book Citation Index
in Web of Science™ Core Collection (BKCI)

Interested in publishing with us?
Contact book.department@intechopen.com

Numbers displayed above are based on latest data collected.
For more information visit www.intechopen.com

For EU product safety concerns:
IN TECH d.o.o., Prolaz Marije Krucifikse Kozulić 3, 51000 Rijeka, Croatia,
info@intechopen.com or visit our website at intechopen.com.

Meet the editor

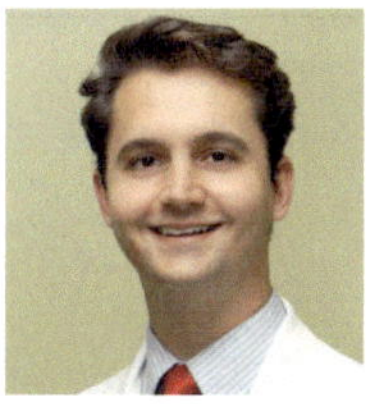

Prof. Fayez Bahmad Jr. is a doctor of medicine and specialist in otology and neurotology. He lives in Brasilia (Brazilian capital). He did the ENT Residency Program at the University of Brasilia Hospital in Otolaryngology between 2002 and 2005 and his PhD degree in the University of Brasilia – Medical School under the orientation of Professor Carlos A. Oliveira, MD, PhD. Professor Oliveira, who has established an otopathology laboratory in his department, is one of the most well-succeeded researchers in otology in Brazil and South America.

He was a member of the Fellowship in Otology and Neurotology at Massachusetts Eye and Ear Infirmary, Harvard Medical School and Fellowship in Human Genetics at Seidman Laboratory, Department of Genetics, Harvard Medical School, when he was engaged in research projects under the mentorship of Professor Saumil N. Merchant, MD, PhD, and Professor Jonathan Seidman, MD, two of the foremost researchers in otology and otopathology and hearing pathogenetics.

He has experience in medicine, focusing on otological surgery, acting on the following subjects: hearing loss and tinnitus. He is the director of the Brasiliense Institute of Otolaryngology, an editor in chief of the traditional *The International Tinnitus Journal,* and a professor at the Faculty of Health Sciences at the University of Brasilia, Brazil.

Contents

Preface

Ménière's disease is an alteration of the inner ear characterized by two groups of symptoms: vestibular symptoms and auditory symptoms. Classical symptoms such as fluctuating hearing loss, tinnitus, atrial fullness, and concomitant dizziness greatly aid the otorhinolaryngologist to diagnose carriers of the disease. But in many patients, their presentation may be different.

In this book, we will adopt the term Ménière's disease to follow the prevailing trend among most research groups and discuss the main topics, current and past ideas about etiopathogenesis, diagnosis, and treatment of Ménière's disease and Ménière's disease associated with migraine.

It is likely that there are genotypic—racial, as well as phenotypic—environmental factors that influence the prevalence difference between countries. One of the major problems in this respect is that the initial presentation of the disease is often the cochlear form, which is not clinically recognized, and is again attributed to another specific cause or is presumed to be simply due to aging. Even after the vestibular component becomes obvious, long periods of remission may mask the complete final image of the syndrome with episodic vertigo, fluctuating autistic loss, tinnitus, and aural fullness. Therefore, generally in clinical practice, only moderate to severe cases are tabulated in the estimates so far.

Some of the epidemiologically published studies to date have tended to blend different epidemiological concepts. The direction of these studies is mainly retrospective (the themes are identified after a result or illness), and they actually measure only prevalence (existing events or the number of cases of a disease at a given moment divided by the population at risk). Only prospective studies (subjects are identified before a result or illness; future events are counted) would have the power to adequately measure this incidence. Although more reflective of real life than an artificial experiment, retrospective observational studies are susceptible to bias.

The multiplicity of diagnostic criteria is another problem that makes it difficult to establish the true incidence of Ménière's disease in the general population. In 1972, the Committee on Hearing and Equilibrium of the American Academy of Otolaryngology-Head and Neck Surgery (AAO-HNS) proposed a specific definition of the disease and guidelines for the evaluation of Ménière in communicating treatment results. In 1985, it was considered that the definition of Ménière's disease needed to be restricted to cases with a complete set of classic signs and symptoms. The 1995 criteria were intended to simplify the definition of Ménière's disease and allow greater flexibility, making it usable in a wide range of studies and classifications. A minimum set of signs and symptoms must be filled in such a way that the degree of certainty of the diagnosis can be established.

Currently, there is no universally accepted theory about the pathophysiology of do-ence. Through histopathological studies, it is presumed that endolymphatic hydrops is the most descriptive pathological characteristic of Ménière's disease. The pathophysiology of the symptoms is still disputed: ruptures of membranes, increased pressure and mechanical displacement of the peripheral organs as the saccule by endolymph accumulation, viral infections, and autoimmune disease in addition to several other theories that have already been reported. It can be seen that in this scheme currently accepted endolymphatic hydrops is no longer a central etiology but rather as one of the manifestations of the syndrome. And the exact mechanism of the etiopathogenesis of the syndrome remains unknown. It is believed that a multifactorial inheritance is the best response, in which the necessary conditions are met to lead to malabsorption of the endolymph and, subsequently, to dropsy. Clinical and laboratory evidence supports this concept.

Dr. Fayez Bahmad Jr
Health Science Faculty of the University of Brasilia
The Brasiliense Institute of Otolaryngology
Brasilia, Brazil

Section 1

Introducton

Chapter 1

Introductory Chapter

Fayez Bahmad

Additional information is available at the end of the chapter

http://dx.doi.org/10.5772/intechopen.69846

Dizziness and vertigo are symptoms related to peripheral vestibular disorders. These are among the most common complaints in medical offices, and knowledge of the major diseases affecting this system is of fundamental importance to the specialist in otolaryngology. In recent years, great advances have been made in otoneurology, which, coupled with increasing knowledge in the field of neurosciences, have substantially modified the approach of the patient with balance complaints. This book studies the most polemic of these vestibular diseases, the Meniere's disease.

Since 2009, the Bárány Society, an international society of otoneurology, has standardized the nomenclature of vestibular symptoms (SV) in four groups: one of the most important is the episodic vestibular syndrome: crises of vestibular symptoms interspersed with asymptomatic periods, such as Menière's syndrome and vestibular migraine [1].

Ménière's disease is an alteration of the inner ear characterized by two groups of symptoms: vestibular symptoms and auditory symptoms. Classical symptoms such as: fluctuating hearing loss, tinnitus, atrial fullness, and concomitant dizziness greatly aid the otorhinolaryngologist to diagnose carriers of the disease. But in many patients, their presentation may be different [1, 2].

The course of the disease may be progressive or nonprogressive, and in addition to the typical clinical presentation of Ménière's disease, two variants of the disease were identified:

1. Meniere's disease Cochlear—symptoms predominantly hearing.
2. Vestibular Ménière's disease—predominantly vestibular symptoms.

And in the literature can still be classified by some authors in two subgroups:

1. Ménière's syndrome symptoms of Ménière's disease caused by a known and well-established condition.
2. Meniere's disease idiopathic cause.

INTECH
open science | open minds

© 2017 The Author(s). Licensee InTech. This chapter is distributed under the terms of the Creative Commons Attribution License (http://creativecommons.org/licenses/by/3.0), which permits unrestricted use, distribution, and reproduction in any medium, provided the original work is properly cited.

In this book, we will adopt the term Ménière's disease to follow the prevailing trend among most research groups and discuss the main topics, current and past ideas about etiopathogenesis, diagnosis, and treatment of Ménière's disease and Ménière's disease associated with migraine.

It is likely that there are genotypic—racial, as well as phenotypic—environmental factors that influence the prevalence difference between countries. One of the major problems in this respect is that the initial presentation of the disease is often the cochlear form, which is not clinically recognized, and is again attributed to another specific cause or is presumed to be simply due to aging. Even after the vestibular component becomes obvious, long periods of re-mission may mask the complete final image of the syndrome with episodic vertigo, fluctuating autistic loss, tinnitus, and aural fullness. Therefore, generally in clinical practice only moderate to severe cases are tabulated in the estimates so far [1–3].

Some of the epidemiologically published studies to date have tended to blend different epidemiological concepts. The direction of these studies is mainly retrospective (the themes are identified after a result or illness), and they actually measure only prevalence (existing events or the number of cases of a disease at a given moment divided by the population at risk). Only prospective studies (subjects are identified before a result or illness, future events are counted) would have the power to adequately measure this incidence. Although more reflective of real life than an artificial experiment, retrospective observational studies are susceptible to bias [4].

Diagnostic failures: The multiplicity of diagnostic criteria is another problem that makes it difficult to establish the true incidence of Ménière's disease in the general population. In 1972, the Committee on Hearing and Equilibrium of the American Academy of Otorhinolaryngology (AAO-HNS) proposed a specific definition of the disease and guidelines for the evaluation of Ménière in communicating treatment results. In 1985, it was considered that the definition of Ménière's disease needed to be restricted to cases with a complete set of classic signs and symptoms. The 1995 criteria were intended to simplify the definition of Ménière's disease and allow greater flexibility, making it usable in a wide range of studies and classifications. A minimum set of signs and symptoms must be filled in such a way that the degree of certainty of the diagnosis can be established [4].

Etiopathogeny: Currently, there is no universally accepted theory about the pathophysiology of do-ence. Through histopathological studies, it is presumed that endolymphatic hydrops is the most descriptive pathological characteristic of Ménière's disease. The pathophysiology of the symptoms is still disputed: ruptures of membranes, increased pressure and mechanical displacement of the peripheral organs as saccule by endolymph accumulation, viral infections, and autoimmune disease in addition to several other theories that have already been reported. It can be seen that in this scheme currently accepted endolymphatic hydrops is no longer a central etiology but rather as one of the manifestations of the syndrome. And the exact mechanism of the etiopathogenesis of the syndrome remains unknown. It is believed that a multifactorial inheritance is the best response, in which the necessary conditions are met to lead to mal absorption of the endolymph and, subsequently, to dropsy. Clinical and laboratory evidence supports this concept [1–4].

http://dx.doi.org/10.5772/intechopen.69846

Author details

Fayez Bahmad

Address all correspondence to: fayezbjr@gmail.com

1 Health Science Faculty of the University of Brasilia, Brasilia, Brazil

2 The Brasiliense Institute of Otolaryngology, Brasilia, Brazil

References

[1] Agrawal Y, Minor LB. Ménière disease and other causes of episodic vertigo. In: Bronstein AM. Vertigo and Imbalance. United Kingdom:Oxford; 2013. pp. 241-250

[2] Bahmad F Jr, DePalma SR, Merchant SN, Bezerra RL, Oliveira CA, Seidman CE, Seidman JG. Locus for familial migrainous vertigo disease maps to chromosome 5q35. The Annals of Otology, Rhinology and Laryngology. 2009 September;**118**(9):670-676

[3] Cal R, Bahmad F Jr. Migraine associated with disfunção auditivo-vestibular auditory-vestibular dysfunction. Brazilian Journal of Otorhinolaryngology. 2008;**74**(4):606-612

[4] Lamounier P, Gobbo DA, de Souza TSA, Bahmad F Jr. Electrocochleography for Ménière's disease: Is it reliable? Brazilian Journal of Otorhinolaryngology. 2014;**80**:527-532

Section 2

Living with Ménière's Disease

Chapter 2

Living with Ménière's Disease: Understanding Patient Experiences of Mental Health and Well-Being in Everyday Life

Jess Tyrrell, Sarah Bell and Cassandra Phoenix

Additional information is available at the end of the chapter

http://dx.doi.org/10.5772/66391

Abstract

This chapter will discuss the current knowledge of the mental health and wellbeing impact of Ménière's. To date, our understanding is limited, with small sample sizes, no controls, and the inability to account for confounding factors. Our work in the UK Biobank aimed to further our understanding of the impacts of Ménière's at the population level.

Secondly we will consider the patient perspective of what it means to live with Ménière's. This is essential to develop appropriate healthcare pathways and ensure patients are able to lead fulfilling lives. There is very limited information about how the patient experiences and makes sense of the disease (or not) - including its triggers and physical sensations - in everyday life.

Our findings suggest that Ménière's adversely impacts on mental health, an individual's emotional state and their life satisfaction. We demonstrate the complex processes of adjustment (physical, social and emotional) following a diagnosis of Ménière's. Although a cure is not currently available, our study illustrates that much can be learnt from the adaptation strategies developed by long-term sufferers in order to help individuals with new diagnoses; an experience that is both daunting and disruptive to patients' everyday lives.

Keywords: Ménière's disease, UK Biobank, Qualitative, mental health, well-being, interdisciplinary

INTECH
open science | open minds

© 2017 The Author(s). Licensee InTech. This chapter is distributed under the terms of the Creative Commons Attribution License (http://creativecommons.org/licenses/by/3.0), which permits unrestricted use, distribution, and reproduction in any medium, provided the original work is properly cited. (cc) BY

1. Introduction

Ménière's disease is a complex multifactorial disorder of the inner ear, consisting of several concurrent symptoms (e.g. aural pressure, hearing loss, tinnitus and vertigo). Patients with Ménière's range from minimally symptomatic highly functional individuals to severely affected disabled patients. Each of the main triad of Ménière's symptoms can impact on quality of life. Tinnitus may be associated with sleep disturbance, depression, irritability, reduced concentration and auditory difficulties [1]. Hearing loss can result in communication difficulties, which can cause problems in work and social life. Vertigo is known to cause anxiety and restrict physical and social activities, therefore significantly impacting on patients' health and well-being [1]. Vertigo is often considered to be the most detrimental and debilitating symptom of Ménière's [2].

Research on the mental health and well-being impact of Ménière's disease is limited. Moreover, quantitative studies in this area are negatively influenced by small sample sizes (often with fewer than 500 participants), a lack of groups to compare the mental health impacts with (i.e. no control groups), and an inability to account for confounding factors. Furthermore, our understanding of how the mental health impact of Ménière's may shift over time is partial at best.

The patient perspective of what it is like to live with this disease within the context of their day-to-day life is critically important for developing appropriate healthcare pathways and ensuring that patients are able to lead as fulfilling lives as possible [3]. While some studies have considered the adverse impact of Ménière's on quality of life, along with patients' perspectives regarding triggers and symptoms of the disease [4], there is very limited information about how patients experience and manage the disease (or not), including its triggers and symptoms in everyday life. In addition, we are currently unaware of the role that other people may play in this process [5–7] or how these issues impact on the sense of mental health and well-being amongst people with Ménière's.

This chapter will build upon existing research in this area, describing a comprehensive, multi-layered two-phase analysis of the impact of Ménière's on patients' mental health and well-being. First, epidemiological analysis from the most powerful Ménière's resource currently available (the UK Biobank, www.biobank.ac.uk) will provide insights on the mental health and well-being impacts of Ménière's at a population level (Phase I). Secondly, qualitative research (Phase II) will provide deeper insights into patients' experiences of living with and negotiating the triggers and symptoms of Ménière's disease on a day-to-day basis, including the role of significant others in this process.

2. Ménière's and mental health at the population level

In Phase I, the UK Biobank dataset was utilised to understand how Ménière's influences mental health and well-being at the population level. This study contained 1376 individuals with self-reported Ménière's and included comprehensive phenotypic data (e.g. anthropometric

http://dx.doi.org/10.5772/66391

measures, early life, lifestyle, family history, medical history, general health and well-being and diet). The aim of this population-level research was to investigate whether people with Ménière's have different mental health and subjective well-being than individuals without the condition. The impact of disease duration on mental health and level of subjective well-being was also investigated within cases.

2.1. Phase I methods

2.1.1. The UK Biobank, Ménière's diagnosis and mental health

The UK Biobank is a phenotypically rich study of over 500,000 individuals aged between 37 and 73 years in 2006–2010 [8]. All participants were interviewed by a nurse, who collated a list of health conditions for each participant. There were several options for ear/vestibular disorders, including tinnitus, vertigo, labyrinthitis, Ménière's disease, otosclerosis or a generic ear/vestibular disorder. The 1376 individuals who reported symptoms of Ménière's disease were selected. An investigation of prescribed medications and key symptom data (e.g. tinnitus and hearing loss) was utilised to validate the variable. For each individual reporting Ménière's, an age of diagnosis was also available and this was utilised to determine disease duration.

The UK Biobank incorporated extensive questions on mental health and subjective well-being. A subsection of questions asked participants to record the frequency of depressed mood, unenthusiasm, tiredness and tenseness within the 2 weeks prior to recruitment. Further questions focused on the number and duration of depression episodes over each participant's life. Participants rated their overall happiness and their satisfaction with health, work, friends and family and finances to provide a range of measures of subjective well-being. Participants were also asked to complete the Eysenck Personality Inventory (EPI) [9].

The participants also reported regular prescription medications, and use of the major antidepressant class—the selective serotonin reuptake inhibitors (SSRIs)—was monitored.

2.1.2. Statistical analysis

The mental health impact of individuals with Ménière's was compared to the whole control population of non-Ménière's sufferers. Linear regression models were utilised to investigate whether a diagnosis of Ménière's influenced the frequency of depression, tiredness, tenseness or unenthusiasm experienced in the 2 weeks prior to recruitment. Similar models were utilised to: (a) investigate how Ménière's influenced subjective well-being; (b) compare the frequency of family contact for cases and controls; and (c) examine the longest duration of depression in cases and controls.

Logistic regression models were used to investigate the odds of: (a) reporting depression; (b) reporting an episode of depression lasting over a week; and (c) utilising SSRIs in Ménière's cases compared to controls.

The role of disease duration on mental health and well-being was investigated. Individuals diagnosed for 5 or more years were compared to those diagnosed within the past 5 years.

Models were adjusted for potential confounders, including participants' age, sex, socio-economic status, waist circumference, home location (urban versus rural as defined by the UK Biobank using the participant's postcodes and the 2001 census data) and ethnicity as covariates. Further adjustment for tinnitus severity was carried out to determine whether this symptom significantly contributed to any mental health associations. Personality is one of the biggest predictors of happiness [10] and therefore the EPI was included as a covariate in the statistical models. All analyses were conducted using STATA/SE Version 12.1 (College Station, USA). Statistical significance was denoted by $P < 0.05$ unless otherwise stated; Bonferroni correction methodology was utilised where appropriate.

2.2. Phase I results

The demographics of the 1376 Ménière's cases and controls are summarised in **Table 1**. As noted in previous studies, there was a preponderance of females (62% versus 54%). The data suggested that individuals with Ménière's had higher proportions of disability benefit than controls (5.3% versus 2.2%, $P < 0.001$) and were more likely to hold disabled badges than controls (8.7% versus 3.6%, $P < 0.001$). Ménière's cases were more likely to be unable to work

Demographics	**All MD sufferers**	**All controls**
N	1376	501,306
Sex		
Male (%)	517 (37.6)	228,677 (45.6)
Female (%)	859 (62.4)	272,629 (54.4)
Mean age at recruitment in years (95% CI)	63.4 (63.0–63.8)	60.4 (60.4–60.5)
Ethnicity (%)		
White	1333 (96.9)	471,525 (94.1)
Mixed	7 (0.5)	2951 (0.6)
Asian	14 (1.0)	9869 (2.0)
Black	2 (0.1)	8065 (1.6)
Chinese	2 (0.1)	1572 (0.3)
Other	7 (0.5)	4554 (0.9)
Missing/unknown	11 (0.8)	2770 (0.5)
Household income		
Less than £18,000	351 (25.5)	96,874 (19.3)
£18,000–£30,999	319 (23.2)	107,891 (21.5)
£31,000–£51,999	250 (18.2)	110,546 (22.0)
£52,000–£100,000	171 (12.4)	86,124 (17.2)
More than £100,000	34 (2.5)	22,900 (4.6)
Missing/unknown	251 (18.2)	76,971 (15.4)

http://dx.doi.org/10.5772/66391

Demographics	All MD sufferers	All controls
Home location		
Urban	1154 (83.9)	427,775 (85.3)
Rural	222 (16.1)	73,513 (14.7)
Disability benefit		
None	1155 (85.5)	465,963 (94.0)
Attendance	6 (0.5)	1150 (0.2)
Disability benefit	72 (5.3)	10,810 (2.2)
Blue badge holder	118 (8.7)	17,871 (3.6)
Employment		
None	8 (0.6)	2795 (0.6)
Employed or self-employed	534 (39.0)	265,185 (53.2)
Retired	588 (43.0)	160,550 (32.2)
Look after home	50 (3.7)	20,032 (4.0)
Don't work because of illness	101 (7.4)	18,940 (3.8)
Unemployed	16 (1.2)	8817 (1.8)
Voluntary	62 (4.5)	17,481 (3.5)
Student	9 (0.7)	4553 (0.9)

Table 1. Demographics of the 1376 Ménière's sufferers and the 501,306 controls in the UK Biobank.

because of illness (7.4% versus 3.8%, χ^2 $P < 0.001$), although it should be noted that the large majority of individuals did work.

2.2.1. Depression

Participants with Ménière's were at higher odds of reporting:

Doctor diagnosed depression odds ratio (OR): 1.53 (95% confidence intervals (CI) 1.32, 1.70, $P < 0.001$, **Figure 1**).

A week long period of depression (OR: 1.33; 95% CI: 1.07, 1.65; $P = 0.011$).

The use of SSRIs (OR: 1.32; 95% CI: 1.01, 1.71; $P = 0.041$).

Ménière's was associated with longer durations of depression—on average this was 10 weeks longer than controls (95% CI: 5.2, 15.2, $P < 0.001$, **Figure 1**).

2.2.2. Mental health impact

Ménière's was associated with increased frequency of depression, tiredness, tenseness and unenthusiasm in the 2 weeks prior to recruitment, although adjustment for the participant's

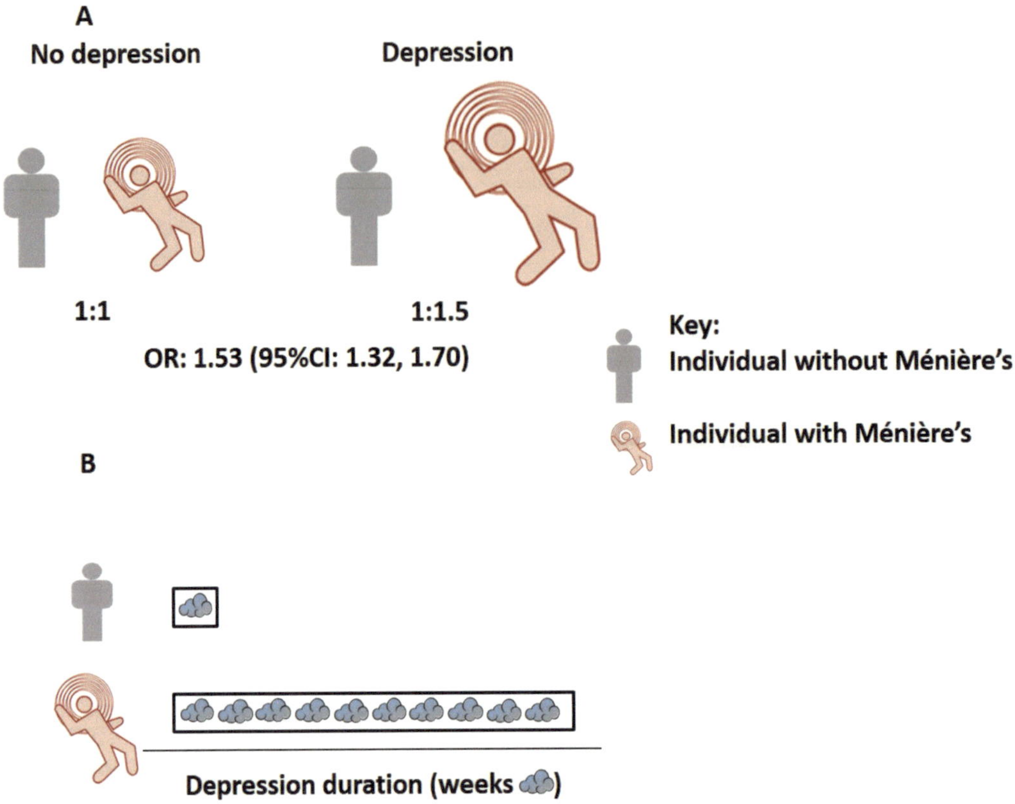

Figure 1. Graphic demonstrating the association between Ménière's and (A) depression and (B) the duration of depression.

neuroticism subscale of the EPI attenuated the regression coefficients with only tiredness remaining significant (**Figure 2**).

Tinnitus, a major symptom of Meniere's, is linked to mental health. Adjustment for tinnitus severity in a subset of the population (n = 168,341), with a similar prevalence of Ménière's (0.25% versus 0.27%), attenuated all the mental health associations.

2.2.3. *Subjective well-being*

Individuals with Ménière's had lower health satisfaction scores than controls and were on average less happy overall. However, there was no difference between cases and controls in terms of satisfaction with their family relationships, friendships and financial situation (**Figure 3**). Higher odds of having social interaction with family and friends on a daily basis (odds ratio 1.5; 95% CI: 1.3, 1.8, $P < 0.001$) or 2–4 times per week (1.2; 1.0, 1.4, $P < 0.01$) was noted for Ménière's cases when compared to controls. The frequency of social interaction predicted individual satisfaction with friends and family.

http://dx.doi.org/10.5772/66391

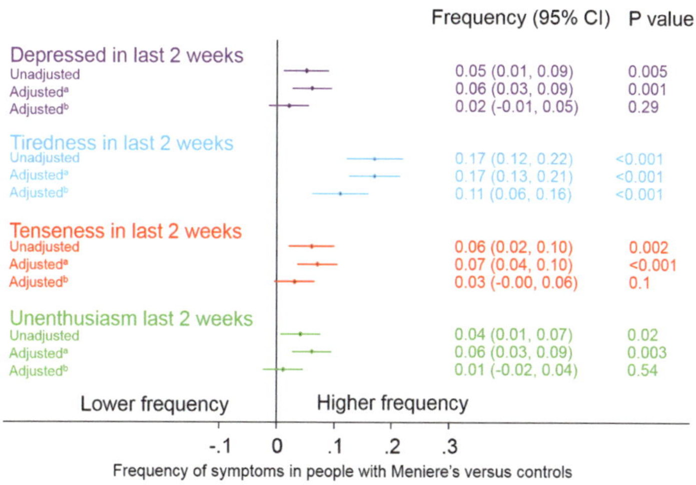

Figure 2. Change in frequency of depression, tiredness, tenseness and unenthusiasm in cases compared to controls. Adjusted[a] accounts for common covariates and Adjusted[b] includes the EPI.

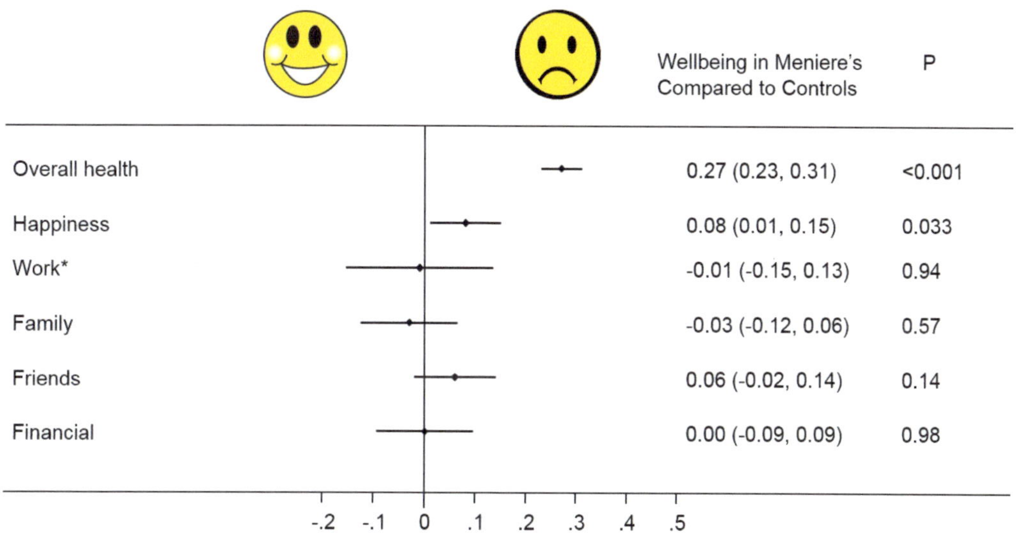

Figure 3. Differences in well-being in cases and controls. *Work satisfaction only asked in individuals with a job.

2.2.4. Disease duration

Within the Ménière's cohort, disease duration was associated with lower levels of depression in the 2 weeks prior to recruitment ($P < 0.05$). Furthermore, individuals diagnosed for more than 5 years were at lower odds of visiting a doctor about depression 0.60 (0.41, 0.90) than recently diagnosed individuals. Longer disease duration was also associated with improved health satisfaction ($P < 0.01$, **Figure 4**).

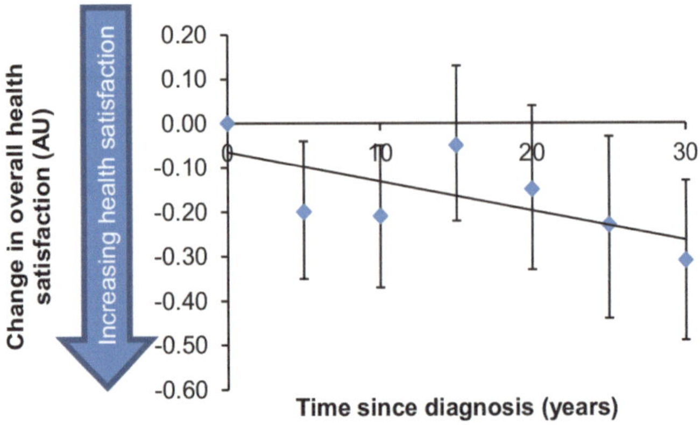

Figure 4. Scatter plot representing how health satisfaction within the Ménière's sufferers changes with time since diagnosis. Regression analysis indicated a significant relationship between overall health satisfaction and disease duration ($P<0.01$).

3. Ménière's and mental health at the individual level

Complementing the population-level analyses, Phase II adopted an in-depth qualitative approach to understand and contextualise people's experiences of Ménière's in their everyday lives. Ethical approval for this phase of the study was secured from the University of Exeter Medical School Research Ethics Committee (Approval Reference 13/09/029).

3.1. Phase II method

With the assistance of the Ménière's Society UK, a purposive sample of 20 Ménière's patients was recruited from across south west England, focusing on individuals diagnosed by an Ear Nose and Throat consultant, reporting symptoms within the previous 12 months (see **Table 2** for sample composition). Purposive sampling allowed information-rich views to be shared by individuals at different stages of the condition, offering insights into the variability of the condition rather than focusing only on the 'typical' or average case [11]. Four participants requested that their partners be present during their interviews, offering emotional support and also providing valuable perspectives on the shared effort of managing and adapting to the onset and progression of Ménière's [12]. A further eight semi-structured interviews were undertaken with partners of other participants to examine these shared and relational impacts in more detail.

Data collection commenced in June 2015, with interviews lasting between 1 and 3.5 hours, all conducted at a time and place of participants' choosing. A flexible interview guide was developed to inform the interview process, using open questions and active listening techniques to facilitate participant-led, open-ended responses. All of the interviews began by giving participants an opportunity to reflect (in their own words) on what was happening in their lives when they first started experiencing symptoms and how things had progressed from there. Follow-up questions focused on: participant interpretations, perceptions of their everyday experiences of the condition; the perceived impacts of the condition on their mental health,

Pseudonym	Age bracket (yrs)	Ménière's duration	Unilateral/bilateral symptoms?	Employment status	Presence of others during interview?
Participants with Ménière's					
Maggie	51–60	<5 yrs	Unilateral	Full time	–
Nicola	31–40	<5 yrs	Unilateral	Full time	–
Jane	61–70	<5 yrs	Unilateral	Retired	–
Louisa	51–60	<5 yrs	Unilateral	Full time	–
Susan	61–70	<5 yrs	Unilateral	Retired	–
Melissa	31–40	<5 yrs	Unilateral	Full time	–
Tom	41–50	<5 yrs	Unilateral	Full time	–
Debbie	61–70	>5 yrs	Unilateral	Non-working	Husband (Mick)
Becky	31–40	>5 yrs	Bilateral	Non-working	Daughter (toddler)
Dawn	51–60	>5 yrs	Unilateral	Early retirement	–
Angus	61–70	>5 yrs	Bilateral	Early retirement	–
Chloe	51–60	>5 yrs	Unilateral	Part time	–
Yvonne	61–70	>5 yrs	Unilateral	Early retirement	–
Caroline	51–60	>5 yrs	Shifting to bilateral	Nonworking	Husband for last half hour
Jennie	41–50	>5 yrs	Bilateral	Part time	Teenage daughter for last half hour
Emily	51–60	>5 yrs	Unilateral	Nonworking	Husband, teenage daughter
Richard	61–70	>5 yrs	Unilateral	Retired	–
Elaine	71–80	>5 yrs	Unilateral	Retired	Husband
John	71–80	>5 yrs	Unilateral	Early retirement	Grandson (periodically through interview)
Emma	51–60	>5 yrs	Unilateral	Self-employed	–
Participants supporting someone with Ménière's					
Karen	62–70	N/A	N/A	Full time	–
David	61–70	N/A	N/A	Self-employed	–
Magda	61–70	N/A	N/A	Part time	–
Matt	61–70	N/A	N/A	Self-employed	-
Sandy	61–70	N/A	N/A	Retired	Wife (Dawn) for last half hour
Mick	71–80	N/A	N/A	Retired	Wife (Debbie)
Toby	51–60	N/A	N/A	Full time	–
Tessa	41–50	N/A	N/A	Part time	Daughter (toddler)

Table 2. Sample composition for the qualitative study.

social roles and identities, friendships and relationships; interactions with the medical profession; the mechanisms by which they tried to self-manage and adapt to the condition over time; and the role of social support in this process.

Interview transcripts were anonymised, checked against the original interview recordings and copies sent back to participants for member-checking purposes [13]. After a period of data immersion, listening back to recordings and annotating transcripts with initial codes and themes, a copy of each transcript and an initial thematic coding framework were uploaded to NVivo 10 (qualitative data management software). Each transcript was then subject to further thematic narrative analysis [14], with the aim of situating emerging themes within each participant's life story, and identifying more subtle, intersecting themes within the data [15]. In order to ensure the analysis and interpretations resonated with individuals living with Ménière's, the early findings were shared and discussed with members of a Ménière's support group in August 2015.

3.2. Phase II results

A key aim of Phase II was to understand more about the adverse mental health impacts observed with the onset and progression of Ménière's, and how participants experienced and negotiated these impacts during their everyday lives. We explore this further in what follows, focusing particularly on the strategies used to adapt to a life of uncertainty in the face of Ménière's, and the roles of supportive partners, family and friends in this process.

Recurring throughout participants' narratives were anxieties linked to the sudden onset of symptoms (vertigo in particular), their varying severity and the unpredictable progression of the condition [16–18]. The accumulation of these anxieties over time resulted in a significant loss of confidence, independence and a deep sense of frustration amongst participants, who likened it to 'driving a car with a dodgy break' and serving a 'prison sentence' with no clear release date. Given the limited efficacy of medication or surgery in treating the condition, participants (and their families) felt powerless in many respects, with even long-term sufferers describing it as 'an alien being' sitting in the body. Throughout participants' interviews, it was apparent that the process of adjusting to life with Ménière's was experienced as a steep and emotionally challenging learning curve, often requiring significant compromises to everyday practices and pleasures.

Participants described lifestyle shifts made in an effort to regain some semblance of control over Ménière's, be they diet-related, or focused more on physical activity, rest and relaxation. Some of these were in response to recommendations from their Ear Nose and Throat consultants (e.g. reducing salt, caffeine and alcohol), whereas others were strategies they had identified through trial and error in the process of learning to 'read' their body as the condition progressed. These included, for example, the use of specific vitamin supplements, postural adjustments, finding activities that would build their core strength without aggravating symptoms (e.g. modified versions of yoga, pilates, tai chi) and maximising sleep and rest where possible. However, participants warned against being overly simplistic in drawing links between stress, relaxation and vertigo severity. Many identified occasions when they had been under significant stress and not had a vertigo attack, or at their most relaxed and still had an attack. As such, although participants engaged in efforts to minimise stress and maximise opportunities for rest and relaxation, they indicated these stress pathways to be complex, inconsistent and intertwined with other factors going on in their lives at the time.

Managing anxiety was highlighted as particularly challenging, even amongst those who had lived with the condition for over 10 years, with many describing a 'shrinking world', loss of spontaneity and sense of isolation. While participants perceived varied potential in counselling, cognitive behavioural therapy and mindfulness interventions, many called for improved access to tailored psychological support from therapists able to appreciate and work with the tangible physical underpinnings of their anxieties. Some conveyed a 'ride the storm' mentality, combining determination with careful contingency strategies in order to cope with the unpredictability of the condition. These participants often described strategies used to distract themselves during less acute, but nonetheless destabilising, stages of an attack, be it watching the clouds through the bedroom window, listening to the radio or taking comfort from the companionship of a quiet cat or dog (reflecting wider literature on the value of companion animals in coping with long-term chronic illness [19, 20]).

> **Debbie:** *'I find having a dog helps, especially this one... I find that touching her does make me feel better... it makes me feel like life's worth living really... She lays still – if she was jumping about I wouldn't be able to stand it, but she seems to sense when I'm not very well and she stays so close to me and still that it does make a difference'.*

Contingency strategies ranged from keeping anti-sickness medication in every pocket/bag, carrying sick bags, tissues, a torch (in winter with shorter hours of daylight), using ear defenders (in noisy settings), wearing sunglasses (to avoid bright light triggers, particularly those living with Ménière's and migraine) and wearing a medical bracelet to convey their emergency contact details if out alone. Perhaps the most important contingency strategy discussed by participants was the role of a reliable support network, be it partners, family or friends, as illustrated in the extract from Dawn's interview below.

> **Dawn:** *'You don't ever feel like "Oh I'm better now, I'll move on." Not completely. There's a little, small percentage of you that's thinking, "Am I going to be okay doing this?"... I have to have a back-up plan. Like, my back-up plan now is that I've trained my husband to actually have his mobile phone with him all the time, which is a massive breakthrough, trust me!'*

Once 'rescued' and brought back to the familiarity of home (described by one participant as their 'cave'), participants explained that they preferred to be left alone to ride out the attack, knowing that someone would be there if needed. In part, this links to feelings of social embarrassment about one's physical state during an attack, but also to the sense that others cannot do much to help at that stage anyway. The increased reliance on partners, family and friends to fulfil this support role was upsetting for some participants, particularly when they felt their condition was compromising the independence of others as well as their own. As one partner commented (the husband of a participant with long-term Ménière's), 'it's not a disease one person gets – if it's a couple, it's a disease that two people get'. Participants, including those with Ménière's and the partners interviewed, explained the need to find a balance between being stoic whilst also recognising limitations. This is illustrated in the extract from Toby's interview below (husband of a participant trying to adapt to bilateral Ménière's).

Toby: *'I mean she probably thinks it's bothered me more than it actually has. The bit that bothers me is to see her suffering. I don't care that I can't go to a pub or cinema… I really don't care about that. She's very stoic, I say this to people – she wouldn't have any gas and air when she had the children. She's a right little tough nut… I mean she won't let it beat her. She'll just, you know, she'll do different-, we'll just do different things'.*

In this extract, Toby draws on an earlier biographical experience (childbirth) to emphasise and show respect for his wife's strength and determination, noting the shared process of finding alternative activities to do together that better accommodate the needs of the condition. Although this was recognised as difficult in particularly active phases of vertigo, several participants described positive examples, including going on outdoor walks, finding quiet pubs/restaurants for lunch or dinner (sitting outside weather-permitting or eating early indoors to avoid crowds and noise), people watching by the coast and visiting nature-based/heritage attractions at quiet times of the day/year. Although this process of finding compensations—be it alone or with a partner, family or friends—often took time, it was deemed particularly important amongst longer-term sufferers:

Emma: *'With the gap that's created by perhaps not being able to do what you would normally do, try and fill it with something else that brings you happiness and pleasure… I've done loads of sewing… and I make these little bags – this is my therapy – I like to have something to show for my day… I've chosen fabrics which are nice and tactile, and in fact I've got a delivery coming today of really amazing bright coloured velvets with velvet silk!'*

Finding these personal 'havens' [21] sometimes required significant (and ongoing) shifts in aspirations and outlook over time, with participants coming to value pleasures and activities they had previously taken for granted. This is indicated in the interview extract below from a participant who had lived with severe symptoms for over 12 years:

Emily: *'I was sort of going along, going along, going along, going along, and then somewhere along this path, I thought "Hang on, we don't do anything. I haven't got a life". I, I, I existed, but I hadn't got a life… But now we have found little places where we can go, so we have got a bit of a life now'.*

The importance of 'counting blessings' came through as particularly important in the interviews of longer-term sufferers. Participants talked about trying to focus on the 'good' things in their lives, making the most of remission phases and cherishing the support networks they have in place to co-navigate the condition. This is conveyed in the extract from Becky's interview below; Becky had lived with Ménière's since she was 17 years old. In her early thirties at the time of the interview, and having recently become a parent, she described the changes in her attitude to the condition since starting to experience bilateral symptoms of tinnitus and imbalance:

Becky: *'I've changed so much in how I've dealt with it. Because before I would have been like, "Oh just get on with it!" to other Ménière's people, you know, "I did". But now I completely understand how devastating an illness it can be… So I just, I'm grateful for each day of normality… I still appreciate living in the now, and living when like my balance is good, and my hearing is good, and the tinnitus isn't so bad… just very much, counting my blessings… focusing on what's good rather than what might happen'.*

Several participants used hope to maintain a sense of morale during the most challenging phases of the condition, particularly with regards to the potential for future medical and technological advances (e.g. stem cells, refined hearing aid and directional microphone technology, etc.) to bring greater understanding of, and predictability to, their condition. Indeed, two participants expressed a reluctance to undergo any of the (albeit limited) surgical procedures currently available for fear of compromising their eligibility for any better, more appealing options emerging further down the line. This touches on the recognition in the wider long-term illness literature that 'absolute faith in medicine may be problematic, prohibit change and be constraining to live by' [22]. As such, it seems important for participants to find a balance between taking comfort from those hopes while also allowing themselves to use all the resources available in the present to fully accept and adapt to their current situation.

4. Discussion

Our research demonstrates that the unpredictable and disabling symptoms of Ménière's result in sufferers experiencing prolonged periods of depression. In addition, it provides insight into how this is experienced in the context of everyday life. We strengthen and extend the evidence from a number of studies suggesting the adverse mental health impact of Ménière's [1, 2, 23], while also supporting previous evidence regarding the impact of Ménière's on fatigue, tenseness and unenthusiasm [23]. The importance of tinnitus severity and mental health outcomes was also highlighted.

Ménière's was strongly associated with lower health status satisfaction. This was unsurprising given the unpredictable nature of the condition and the known association with depression. Indeed, many of our participants lived with an ongoing sense of anxiety as symptoms caused their body to 'dys-appear', or emerge problematically into direct consciousness [24]. Moreover, this occurred in ways that were not only unpredictable but also uncontrollable. Losing control over a body that, prior to the onset of symptoms (severe or otherwise), had become disciplined and predictable through acts of routinised self-regimentation (working, exercising, eating, socialising and so forth—without the need for careful and strategic planning) further contributed to mental distress [25].

The similarity in other life domains between people with Ménière's and controls, including satisfaction with family, friends and financial status, is particularly noteworthy. It might be anticipated that because of their condition people with Ménière's would be less satisfied with all aspects of their life. However, previous work on other chronic health conditions has suggested that people do not always rate their quality of life as badly as healthy people might anticipate [26]. Further some studies have demonstrated small differences in reported life satisfaction or happiness between people with serious physical disabilities and 'normal' control subjects [27]. One explanation for this might be found in our participants' accounts of learning to find joy and happiness in activities that formed the fabric of their daily life, but had previously been taken for granted. Included here was the realisation of unwavering support and in some instances, new found closeness with the people around them. Indeed, the data suggested that individuals with Ménière's had more contact and satisfactory relationships with family and friends.

In day-to-day life, people with Ménière's can feel isolated, afraid, dependent and on some occasions embarrassed. Yet, reflecting previous literature on chronic illness [21], our research highlights the value of support networks and suggests they may enable people with Ménière's to live satisfying lives. We would, therefore, emphasise the importance of not just informing friends and family about the condition, but educating them on how they might best assist during its various manifestations. This might range from being mindful of inclusive forms of communication for those with impaired hearing, to supporting from afar during an attack. Aasbo et al.'s [28] concept of 'biographical we' is useful here in helping to understand the great effort partners of chronically ill put in to re-establish normality and continuity in everyday life; effort, that as our research signalled, can come at a cost of their own needs being overlooked. 'Ménière's is a disease that two people get' and this aspect warrants greater consideration as part of the broader patient treatment pathway.

Improvements in the frequency of depression episodes and health satisfaction were noted as disease duration increased. This may reflect the disease progression pathway, which usually involves a reduction in the number of vertigo attacks experienced by individuals as the disease progresses [29]. Our participants' improved ability to read their bodies and recognise signs of an impending attack suggests the development of *Ménière's literacy*. Borrowing from the concept of *interactive health literacy*, whereby individuals develop an improved capacity to act independently on knowledge with motivation and confidence in an empowered way [30], *Ménière's literacy supports* adaptation by individuals to their condition and/or medical interventions and lifestyle changes reducing the frequency of vertigo attacks. Given that vertigo is considered to be the most detrimental symptom in Ménière's [2], reductions in vertigo severity should, therefore, improve mental health and well-being. All of this is not to suggest that adaptation diminishes the ongoing sensory, emotional and social challenges that people with Ménière's face in their everyday life [16]. Indeed, our research showed that at a population level, disease duration did not alter the frequency of tiredness, tenseness or a lack of enthusiasm experienced by Ménière's sufferers. While some aspects of Ménière's may improve over time and an individual may adapt to some extent, overall it continues to impact negatively on everyday life.

5. Conclusions

Our research findings emerged from cross-sectional data. It cannot and does not seek to determine the causal pathway of Ménière's disease. Our interpretations of the qualitative data are shaped as much by the absence of certain voices as they are by the presence of others. To that end, it is noteworthy that our sample for Phase II consisted primarily of women (16 female patients, 3 female supportive partners), with just four participants experiencing bilateral symptoms of tinnitus, imbalance and hearing loss (i.e. symptoms in both ears).

Those limitations noted, the research provides the most comprehensive study of the mental health and well-being impacts of Ménière's to date and highlights the adverse mental health effects of Ménière's. By utilising the UK Biobank, the inclusion of key confounders and sufficient numbers to investigate the role of disease duration in Phase I has enabled us to offer a unique contribution to the field. Likewise, a combined focus on the individual everyday realities of living with Ménière's disease provides original insight into how it intersects with mental health and well-being in a number of different ways and across a variety of contexts. While offering a holistic and detailed analysis of this subject, the research also provides a working example of interdisciplinary, integrated research and the value it can bring to our attempts to understand complex health conditions like Ménière's disease in a way that respects the importance of the big picture, without ignoring the individual 'expert' voices of patient experience.

Acknowledgements

The research presented in this book chapter was funded by the UK Ménière's Society. The Phase I research was conducted using the UK Biobank resource. We would like to thank participants from the UK Biobank and those that took part in the Phase II research.

Author details

Jess Tyrrell[1]*, Sarah Bell[1] and Cassandra Phoenix[2]

*Address all correspondence to: j.tyrrell@exeter.ac.uk

[1] University of Exeter, Exeter, United Kingdom

[2] University of Bath, Bath, United Kingdom

References

[1] Yardley L, Dibb B, Osborne G. Factors associated with quality of life in Meniere's disease. Clinical Otolaryngology and Allied Sciences. 2003;28(5):436-41.

[2] Arroll M, Dancey CP, Attree EA, Smith S, James T. People with symptoms of Meniere's disease: the relationship between illness intrusiveness, illness uncertainty, dizziness handicap, and depression. Otology and Neurotology. 2012;33(5):816-23.

[3] Paterson C, Britten N. Organising primary health care for people with asthma: the patient's perspective. The British Journal of General Practice : the Journal of the Royal College of General Practitioners. 2000;50(453):299-303.

[4] Kirby SE, Yardley L. Physical and psychological triggers for attacks in Meniere's disease: the patient perspective. Psychotherapy and Psychosomatics. 2012;81(6):396-8.

[5] Manchaiah VK, Pyykko I, Kentala E, Levo H, Stephens D. Positive impact of Meniere's disorder on significant others as well as on patients: our experience from eighty-eight respondents. Clinical Otolaryngology. 2013;38(6):550-4.

[6] Pyykko I, Nakashima T, Yoshida T, Zou J, Naganawa S. Meniere's disease: a reappraisal supported by a variable latency of symptoms and the MRI visualisation of endolymphatic hydrops. BMJ Open. 2013;3(2). Pii: e001555.

[7] Stephens D, Pyykko I, Kentala E, Levo H, Rasku J. The effects of Meniere's disorder on the patient's significant others. International Journal of Audiology. 2012;51(12):858-63.

[8] Collins R. What makes UK Biobank special? Lancet. 2012;379(9822):1173-4.

[9] Eysenck HJ, Eysenck SBG. Manual of Eysenck Personality Inventory. London: University of London Press; 1964.

[10] DeNeve KM, Cooper H. The happy personality: a meta-analysis of 137 personality traits and subjective well-being. Psychological Bulletin. 1998;124(2):197-229.

[11] Flyvbjerg B. Five misunderstandings about case study research. Qualitative Inquiry. 2006;12:219-45.

[12] Polak L, Green J. Using joint interviews to add analytic value. Qualitative Health Research. 2015;26(12):1638-48.

[13] Sparkes AC, Smith B. Qualitative Research Methods in Sport, Exercise and Health: From Process to Product. Abingdon: Routledge; 2014.

[14] Riessman CK. Narrative Methods for the Human Sciences. London: SAGE Publications Ltd.; 2008.

[15] Phoenix C, Smith B, Sparkes AC. Narrative analysis in aging studies: a typology for consideration. Journal of Aging Studies. 2010;24(1):1-11.

[16] Bell SL. The role of fluctuating soundscapes in shaping the emotional geographies of individuals living with Meniere's Disease. Social & Cultural Geography. 2016: 1-20.

[17] Bell SL, Tyrrell J, Phoenix C. A day in the life of Meniere's disease. Sociology of Health and Illness. 2016 In Press.

[18] Bell SL, Tyrrell J, Phoenix C. Ménière's disease and biographical disruption: Where family transitions collide. Social Science & Medicine. 2016 (166):177-85

[19] Brooks HL, Rogers A, Kapadia D, Pilgrim J, Reeves D, Vassilev I. Creature comforts: personal communities, pets and the work of managing a long-term condition. Chronic Illness. 2013;9(2):87-102.

[20] Ryan S, Ziebland S. On interviewing people with pets: reflections from qualitative research on people with long-term conditions. Sociology of Health and Illness. 2015;37(1):67-80.

[21] Lundman B, Jansson L. The meaning of living with a long-term disease. To revalue and be revalued. Journal of Clinical Nursing. 2007;16(7B):109-15.

[22] Smith B, Sparkes AC. Men, sport, spinal cord injury, and narratives of hope. Social Science & Medicine. 2005;61(5):1095-105.

[23] Levo H, Stephens D, Poe D, Kentala E, Pyykko I. Use of ICF in assessing the effects of Meniere's disorder on life. Annals of Otology, Rhinology and Laryngology. 2010;119(9):583-9.

[24] Leder D. The Absent Body. Chicago: University of Chicago Press; 1990.

[25] Frank AW. The Wounded Storyteller. Body, Illness and Ethics. Chicago: University of Chicago Press; 1995.

[26] Buick DL, Petrie KJ. "I Know Just How You Feel": The validity of healthy women's perceptions of breast-cancer patients receiving treatment. Journal of Applied Social Psychology. 2002;32(1):110-23.

[27] Riis J, Loewenstein G, Baron J, Jepson C, Fagerlin A, Ubel PA. Ignorance of hedonic adaptation to hemodialysis: a study using ecological momentary assessment. Journal of Experimental Psychology General. 2005;134(1):3-9.

[28] Aasbo G, Solbraekke KN, Kristvik E, Werner A. Between disruption and continuity: challenges in maintaining the 'biographical we' when caring for a partner with a severe, chronic illness. Sociology of Health and Illness. 2016;38(5):782-96.

[29] Huppert D, Strupp M, Brandt T. Long-term course of Meniere's disease revisited. Acta Otolaryngology. 2010;130(6):644-51.

[30] Nutbeam D. Health literacy as a public health goal: a challenge for contemporary health education and communication strategies into the 21st century. Health Promotion International. 2000;15(3):259-67.

Section 3

Ménière's Disease - Epidemiology

Chapter 3

Ménière's Disease: Epidemiology

Liane Sousa Teixeira and
Aliciane Mota Guimarães Cavalcante

Additional information is available at the end of the chapter

http://dx.doi.org/10.5772/intechopen.69666

Abstract

Meniere's disease is a disorder of the membranous labyrinth of the inner ear manifesting as vertigo, tinnitus, sensory neural hearing loss and aural fullness of known or unknown origin. The aim of this chapter is to estimate the prevalence of Ménière's disease (MD) and its relationship with demographic factors, symptoms and conditions that are known. Few articles have been published on the epidemiology of Meniere's disease from 1975 to 1990, studies from Japan indicated a fairly constant prevalence of 17 cases per 100,000 population. These studies were undertaken by a Research Committee on Meniere's Disease. Kotimaki and colleagues analysed the Finnish population of five million people between 1992 and 1996. A prevalence of 43/100,000 and an average yearly incidence of 4.3/100,000 population were found by the authors. MD is 1–3 times higher in women than in men and also observed a higher prevalence in adulthood and white people. MD seems to be much more common in white adults with higher body mass index categories, in their fourth and fifth decade. However, in recent years, especially in the last decades, there have been several safe and effective medical and surgical therapies for the treatment of the disease and its sequels.

Keywords: epidemiology, prevalence, Ménière, incidence, hearing loss

1. Introduction

Symptom and disease definitions are a fundamental prerequisite for professional communication in clinical, research and public health settings. The need for structured criteria for epidemiologic, diagnostic and therapeutic research is more obvious for disciplines that rely heavily on syndromic diagnosis [1].

Accurate information about the occurrence and impact of balance disorders is also important for planning health services that meet the needs of the community they serve. It is essential to have a good understanding of the epidemiology of the conditions and their symptomatic

INTECH
open science | open minds

© 2017 The Author(s). Licensee InTech. This chapter is distributed under the terms of the Creative Commons Attribution License (http://creativecommons.org/licenses/by/3.0), which permits unrestricted use, distribution, and reproduction in any medium, provided the original work is properly cited.

presentation in the community. Much literature in this area is based around specialist clinic and hospital experience that is likely to be subject to bias [2].

The challenge in diagnosing Meniere's disease continues, because usually in the early stages, only a few symptoms are present. Consequently, there is a difficulty in measuring the incidence and prevalence of the disease in any population. In the emergency department, it is common to see patients with Ménière's disease (MD) discharged with inaccurate labyrinthitis dignitaries after sudden onset of vertigo [3].

Ménière's disease is characterised by recurrent attacks of vertigo associated with fluctuating sensorineural hearing loss, tinnitus and a sense of aural fullness. In 1861, Prosper Ménière correctly attributed the attacks to a disorder of the inner ear, suggesting that the mechanism of causation could be similar to migraine or inner ear vasospasm, a differential diagnosis which is still relevant for the disease today [4].

2. Studies review

Few articles have been published on the epidemiology of Meniere's disease [3].

Despite the large number of scientific contributions published annually on Meniere's disease, consistent epidemiologic information is sparse. To date, the true incidence and prevalence of Meniere's disease are not known [5].

Table 1 shows some articles published in the literature and the number of patients in each study presented.

Author	Journal	Year	Subject
Murdin [2]	Otology and Neurotology	2015	Studies were eligible for inclusion if they contained data on the epidemiology of symptoms of balance disorders (dizziness and vertigo) or balance disorders sampled from community-based adult populations. Twenty eligible studies were identified
Simo	American Journal of Otolaryngology	2015	Described the prevalence of Meniere's disease in the United States between 2008 and 2010 in patients >10 years old. Prevalence was highest in Caucasians 91 per 100,000 people
Tyrrell [15]	Ear and Hearing	2014	The aim of this study was to estimate the prevalence of Ménière's disease, which was more common in participants who were older, white, female and having higher body mass index categories. The authors used cross-sectional data from the UK Biobank to compare 1376 self-reported Ménière's participants
Angulo [13]	Acta Otorrinolaringológica Española	2003	We prospectively collected all patients diagnosed with Meniere's disease 'definitive' between 1992 and 2002 Sierrallana Hospital in Torrelavega (Cantabria). The incidence was 3/100,000 cases inhabitants/year prevalence of 75/100,000 (29 in men and 46 in women)
Shojaku [10]	ORL	2005	They conducted retrospective surveys for the period 1990–2004 of the Nishikubiki district and of the period 1980–2004 of Toyama Medical and Pharmaceutical University. The average annual prevalence was 34.5 per 100,000 population

Author	Journal	Year	Subject
Vrabec [7]	Otolaryngology–Head and Neck Surgery	2007	Retrospective review in an academic referral practice. To define the prevalence of definite Ménière's disease (MD) among patients presenting with characteristic symptoms and examine the utility of published diagnostic guidelines. The prevalence of definite MD in these 295 individuals was 64%
Havia [11]	Otolaryngology–Head and Neck Surgery	2005	Prospective study based on population register data to study the prevalence of Menière's disease in the general population of Southern Finland. The prevalence of 513 of 100,000 persons, but our population-based estimate of MD prevalence is much higher than in previous reports

Table 1. Articles published in the literature.

3. Epidemiology

Although Ménière's syndrome (MS) has been recognized as a clinical entity since 1861, when it was first described by Prosper Ménière, the epidemiology of the disorder is still uncertain [6].

In 1861, Prosper Ménière first described the clinical trial that bears his name. The knowledge of cochleovestibular function was primitive. Today, physicians are still grappling with the same questions regarding the pathophysiology of the syndrome that perplexed Ménière 145 years ago, in the age of high-resolution imaging, molecular diagnostics and single-cell physiology [7].

Several epidemiological studies of Ménière's disease have been performed over the past few decades with widely contrasting results. The wide range is likely to result from changes over time in criteria for the diagnosis of Ménière's disease, methodological differences, differences in the populations surveyed and difficulty in distinguishing Ménière's disease from related conditions such as migraine-associated vertigo [8].

Many of the epidemiologic studies have to rely on chart reviews or medical databases, each having their own flaws. Data collected during routine clinical care will vary in quality, and their interpretation is limited by the consistency, accuracy, availability and completeness of source records. Although more reflective of 'real life' than a contrived experiment, observational retrospective studies are susceptible to bias. Although studies of medical databases are relatively inexpensive and data often are already organized and computerized, these studies do not eliminate possible bias, often present high rates of missing data or errors, and have definitions by which data are encoded that may change over time (absolutely true in Meniere's disease) [5].

Published reports of the epidemiology of MS generally fall into two methodological categories. Most published studies are retrospective series that start with known cases of MS identified from patient records for a given group of hospitals and clinics. The population served by the hospitals and clinics then serves as the dominator for calculating incidence and prevalence. This methodology introduces sampling bias in that patients in the population with the disease may not have been treated at the hospitals and clinics surveyed for various reasons. Population-based cross-sectional studies reduce sampling bias by surveying a random sample of the general population [6].

In an effort to improve reporting of disease outcomes and ensure a uniform definition of the disease, the American Academy of Otolaryngology—Head and Neck Surgery (AAO-HNS)

Hearing and Equilibrium Committee has issued guidelines for diagnosis. The most recent version of the guidelines was presented in 1995 [7].

Prevalence is defined as the proportion of individuals in a population having a disease [9].

In 1973, Stahle and colleagues reported a prevalence of 46 cases per 100,000 population. From 1975 to 1990, studies from Japan indicated a fairly constant prevalence of 17 cases per 100,000 population. These studies were undertaken by a Research Committee on Meniere's Disease and a Committee on Peripheral Vestibular Disorders. Kotimaki and colleagues reported a prevalence of 43/100,000 and an average annual incidence of 4/3,000,000 inhabitants after analysing the Finnish population for a period of 4 years according to the AAO-HNS recommendations [3].

The study with the highest number of citations examining prevalence of MS in the United States was performed by Wladislavosky-Waserman and colleagues. These investigators identified cases of MS by examining medical records from 1953 to 1980 for the Mayo Clinic and Olmstead Medical Group, the major healthcare providers for the 40,000 inhabitants of Rochester, Minnesota. A prevalence of 218 per 100,000 in 1980 was reported. As Celestino and Ralli pointed out, one-third of patients included in the Rochester study had recurrent vertigo without cochlear symptoms and would not meet current criteria for MS. Therefore, prevalence was likely overestimated. Also, the population studied was homogeneous relative to the current United States population; 99% of the subjects were white [9].

Estimated prevalence rates range from as low as 3.5 per 100,000 population to as high as 513 per 100,000 population. However, it is clear that Ménière's disease is more common in women [8].

The frequency of male/female prevalence in Meniere's disease has been noted to be generally equal with perhaps some slight female preponderance. Simo et al. described the prevalence of Meniere's disease in the United States. This study clearly provides evidence that currently a female preponderance is present. The findings of a female predominance is 1.51, but not unlike other reported rates of gender differences [4].

Harris also showed the prevalence of Meniere's disease by age group and sex, as shown in **Figure 1**.

A study was conducted to estimate the prevalence of Meniere's disease in the UK. This study investigated the relationship between some conditions such as mental health, diseases and demographic factors.

They used data from the UK Biobank to compare 1376 self-reported Ménière's participants with over 500,000 participants without Ménière's disease.

Ménière's disease was more common in participants who were older, having higher body mass index categories, white and female.

After World War II, to rapid increase in cases of MD occurred in Japan, but the reasons have not yet been clarified.

In Nishikubiki district, a retrospective survey of 15 years was conducted to evaluate epidemiological characteristics, such as sex and age. Some of the data in this study were analysed in a previous study. Three hundred and sixty-five patients were diagnosed with MD according to the diagnostic criteria. There was a slight increase in the prevalence of MD during the period 1990–2004 [10].

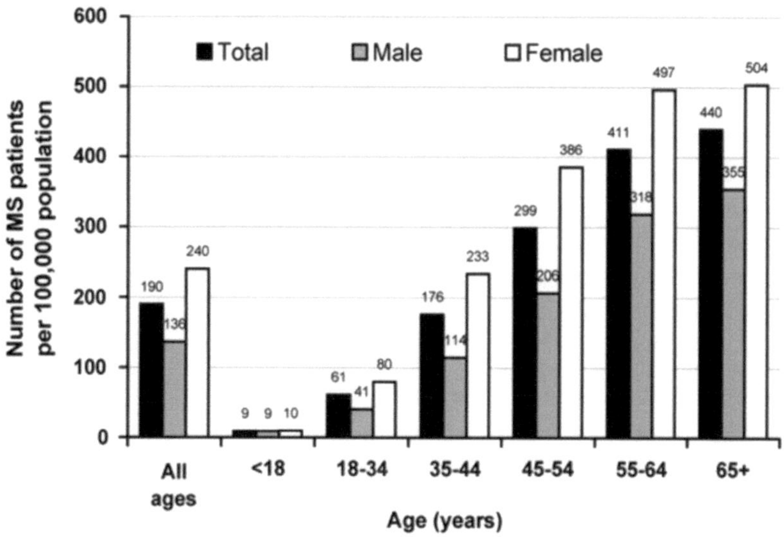

Figure 1. Prevalence in the United States of Meniere's syndrome by age group and sex. From Harris and Alexander [9].

In Houston—TX, a retrospective chart review was conducted to identify outpatient visits coded using the ICD-9 codes for Ménière's disease during the years 2001–2003. The prevalence of definite MD in these 295 individuals was 64%. For this study, the 1995 American Academy of Otolaryngology-Head and Neck Surgery (AAO-HNS) Committee on Hearing and Equilibrium guidelines were used for diagnosis and classification. The largest group (23%) consisted of patients with only cochlear symptoms. Of those with definite MD, the mean duration of disease at last follow-up was 7.6 years, 56% were female, 19% had bilateral disease and 34% required surgical management for vertigo. Those initially classified as probable are usually reclassified as definite with extended follow-up [7].

The prevalence of Menière's disease was evaluated in the general population of Southern Finland through a prospective study based on population register data. A prospective MD prevalence study was conducted in the general population of Southern Finland. A questionnaire on vertigo associated with a sensation of movement, hearing loss or tinnitus was sent to 5000 people from the age of 12 years randomly selected in the city. The patients were clinically examined in our vestibular unit. The clinical examination was supplemented by audiological and otoneurological examinations [11].

The response rate was 63%. In the final sample of 3116 people, 216 reported the triad of vertigo, hearing loss and tinnitus. Using the most recent criteria of the Hearing and Balance Committee of the American Academy of Otorhinolaryngology-Head and Neck Surgery, we were able to identify 16 patients with definite DM of the total sample, obtaining a prevalence of 513 of 100,000 people. Of the 16 patients with MD, nine patients had already been diagnosed with MD and one patient was diagnosed during the clinical examination. A peak prevalence of 1709 of 100,000 was seen in the age range of 61–70 years. However, MD prevalence in Southern Finland is overvalued relative to the rest of the world. However, the MD prevalence in Southern Finland is much higher than the prevalence estimations based on hospital registers around the world as suggested [11].

MD is associated with several comorbid conditions such as arthritis (OR 1.8), psoriasis (OR 1.8), gastroesophageal reflux disease (OR 1.5), irritable bowel syndrome (OR 2.1) and migraine (OR 2.0). The development of cochlear and vestibular symptoms has a variable course and can take years in individual patients [12].

Depending on the series, the male/female ratio varies curiously. Some reports point out that Meniere's disease affects both sexes equally or there is a slight female preponderance, up to 1.3:1. Wladislavosky-Waserman and colleagues reported a slight (though not statistically significant) preponderance of females. Following the three decades covered by the study, there was a progressive decline over time in numbers of women affected. In contrast, for men, there was a slight (but not significant) increase in rates for the same period [5].

Most studies suggest a slight female preponderance of up to 1.3 times that of men. MD seems to be much more common in white adults with higher body mass index categories, in their fourth and fifth decade. However, it can also be observed in children. A prevalence of 3% of MD was observed by Meyerhoff and colleagues in the paediatric population. Many studies have shown the existence of a positive family history for Meniere's disease with an index of relatives affected up to 20%.

The prevalence increases dramatically with age, peaking in the 60–69 years age group. It is very rare in people younger than 20 years [7]. This increase is shown in the graph in **Figure 2**. Already the incidence rate of Meniere's disease by gender according to age groups can be seen in **Figure 3**.

	11-20	21-30	31-40	41-50	51-60	61-70	71-80	81-90	>90
Prevalence (per 100,000)	3	7	23	56	84	100	111	118	110

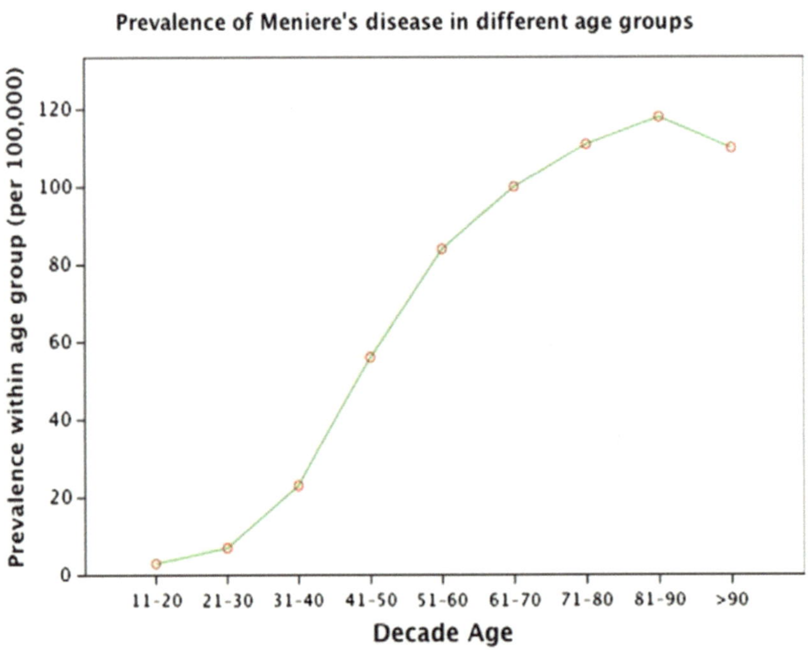

Figure 2. Prevalence of Meniere's disease at different decade age in inpatients population.

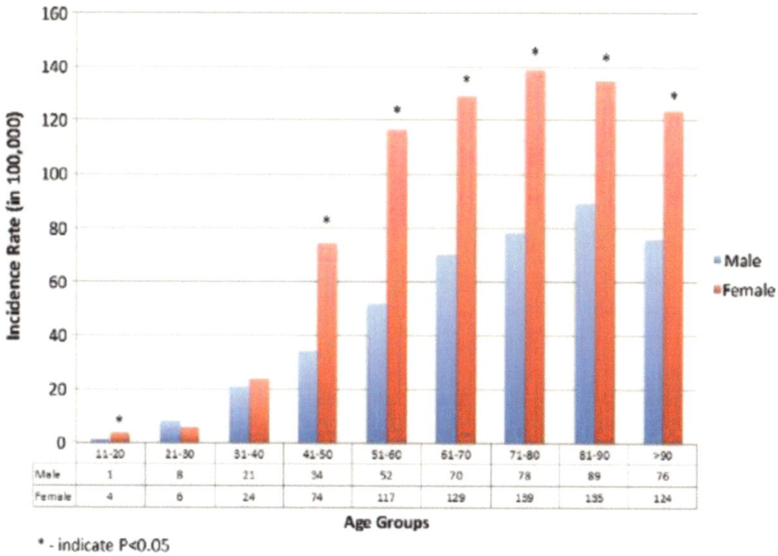

Figure 3. Incidence rate of Meniere's disease by gender according to age groups.

Unfortunately, for disorders such as MS that are relatively rare at the population level, very large sample sizes are needed to achieve sufficient power to accurately estimate epidemiological characteristics in population-based studies [6].

4. Estimates of incidence

Incidence is defined as the number of new cases occurring over a specified period of time, usually 1 year [9]. Incidence rate represents the number of new cases of a disease over a specified period of time divided by the population at risk [5].

The incidence and prevalence in the general population are inferred from the exact values in the sample group [6].

Only prospective studies (subjects are identified prior to an outcome or disease; future events are recorded) have the power to measure incidence [5].

In 1954, Cawthorne and Hewlett attempted to estimate the incidence of MS by examining a register of clinical records for eight clinical practices in Great Britain serving a population of 27,365 people; they arrived at an annual incidence of 157 per 100,000. As pointed out by Wladislavosky-Waserman and colleagues, this number most likely represents a combination of incidence and prevalence, as some patients may have had onset of symptoms in preceding years.

In 1973, Stahle and colleagues examined records from a standard, nationally administered record system to determine the incidence of MS in a patient population from two cities in Sweden; they found an annual incidence of 46 per 100,000. Celestino and Ralli reviewed the records from 1973 to 1985 from a hospital and outpatient clinic serving a community of 1,03,797 people in Italy. The 1972 American Academy of Ophthalmology and Otolaryngology guidelines were applied for diagnosis of MS, and an incidence of 8.2 per 10,00,000 people per year was found [9].

A study in Cantabria evaluated epidemiological data. Incidence was determined by the number of patients diagnosed Meniere's disease with per 100,000 inhabitants/year during the 11 years of the study and residents in the area having a health study excluding Meniere previous diagnosis of disease. The incidence was 3/100,000 cases inhabitants/year prevalence of 75/100,000 (29 in men and 46 in women). The most common age of diagnosis was between 40 and 60 years [13].

In Japan, the average annual incidence was 5.0 per 100,000 population. Incidence and prevalence predominated in females. With respect to age at disease, the incidence in elderly patients was increased when we corrected for age distribution in the overall population [10].

5. Meniere familial

Familial MD should be considered if at least one other relative (first or second degree) fulfills all the criteria of definite or probable MD. Familial MD should be considered if at least one other relative (first or second degree) fulfills all the criteria of definite or probable MD. Familial MD is observed in 8–9% of sporadic cases in populations of European descent. This was also described in Caucasians from Brazil, Sweden, Finland, United Kingdom, Spain and Germany. Although most families described have an autosomal dominant pattern of inheritance, familial MD shows genetic heterogeneity, and mitochondrial and recessive inheritance patterns are also observed in some families [12].

5.1. Associated symptoms

The symptom triad of vertigo, tinnitus and hearing loss all contribute to the disabling nature of the condition. Ménière's disease is an unpredictable illness that affects mental health. Ménière's disease is an unpredictable illness that affects mental health. Tyrrell et al. investigated the mental health of 1376 Ménière's disease patients. Participants answered 38 questions to mental health. They utilized crude and adjusted linear to investigate the association between Ménière's disease and mental health.

Ménière's disease was associated with increased frequency of tenseness, depression, tiredness and unenthusiasm in the 2 weeks before recruitment. Ménière's disease was associated with longer periods of depression than controls. Reduced health satisfaction was associated with Ménière's disease, but in other aspects of life (general happiness, work, family, financial), individuals with Ménière's disease were as happy as controls. Mental health and SWB in individuals diagnosed for longer was better than in those who were recently diagnosed suggesting at least adaptation.

The results show that Ménière's disease has a negative impact on the individual's satisfaction with life, their mental health and emotional state.

These results raise the importance of supporting social relationships, since long-term patient adaptation strategies can help those with new diagnoses. This is the largest population study investigating the mental health impact of Ménière's disease [14].

Author details

Liane Sousa Teixeira[1]* and Aliciane Mota Guimarães Cavalcante[2]

*Address all correspondence to: liane_st21@hotmail.com

1 Brasiliense Institute of Otolaryngology, Health Science Faculty, University of Brasilia Medical School, Brasília, Distrito Federal, Brazil

2 Brasiliense Institute of Otolaryngology, Brasília, Distrito Federal, Brazil

References

[1] Bisdorff, Alexandre R., Jeffrey P. Staab, and David E. Newman-Toker. "Overview of the international classification of vestibular disorders." Neurologic clinics 33.3, 2015: 541-550

[2] Murdin, L., & Schilder, A. G. Epidemiology of balance symptoms and disorders in the community: a systematic review. Otology & Neurotology, 2015, **36**(3), 387-392.

[3] Sajjadi, H., & Paparella, M. M. Meniere's disease. The Lancet, 2008, **372**(9636), 406-414.

[4] Hermann S, BS, Shiayin Y, Weikai Q, Michal P, Munier N, Reginald B, Meniere's disease: importance of socioeconomic and environmental factors, American Journal Otolaryngoloy - Head and Neck Medicine and Surgery 36, 2015, 393-398

[5] da Costa, S. S., de Sousa, L. C. A., & de Toledo Piza, M. R. Meniere's disease: overview, epidemiology, and natural history. Otolaryngologic Clinics of North America, 2002 **35**(3), 455-495

[6] Harris, J. P., & Alexander, T. H. Current-day prevalence of Meniere's syndrome. Audiology and Neurotology, 2010, **15**(5), 318-322

[7] Vrabec, J. T., Simon, L. M., & Coker, N. J. Survey of Ménière's disease in a subspecialty referral practice. Otolaryngology--Head and Neck Surgery, 2007, **137**(2), 213-217.

[8] Melville, D. C. F. Ménière's disease A stepwise approach, MedicineToday; 2014, **15**(3): 18-26

[9] Alexander, T. H., & Harris, J. P. Current epidemiology of Meniere's syndrome. Otolaryngologic Clinics of North America, 2010, **43**(5), 965-970

[10] Shojaku, H., Watanabe, Y., Fujisaka, M., Tsubota, M., Kobayashi, K., Yasumura, S., & Mizukoshi, K. Epidemiologic characteristics of definite Meniere's disease in Japan. ORL, 2005, **67**(5), 305-309

[11] Havia, M., Kentala, E., & Pyykkö, I. Prevalence of Meniere's disease in general population of Southern Finland. Otolaryngology-Head and Neck Surgery, 2005, **133**(5), 762-768

[12] Lopez-Escamez, J. A., Carey, J., Chung, W. H., Goebel, J. A., Magnusson, M., Mandalà, M., ... & Bisdorff, A. Diagnostic criteria for Menière's disease. Journal of Vestibular Research, 25(1), 1-7.Melville da Cruz Fracs, Ménière's disease A stepwise approach, MedicineToday 2014; **15**(3): 18-26

[13] Angulo, C. M., Castellanos, R. G., Mantilla, J. G., Capelastegui, J. B., & Carrera, F. Epidemiología de la Enfermedad de Meniere en Cantabria. Acta Otorrinolaringológica Española, 2003, **54**(9), 601-605.

[14] Tyrrell, J., White, M. P., Barrett, G., Ronan, N., Phoenix, C., Whinney, D. J., & Osborne, N. J. Mental health and Subjective well-being of individuals with Meniere's: cross-sectional analysis in the UK biobank. Otology & Neurotology, 2015, **36**(5), 854-861.

[15] Tyrrell, J. S., Whinney, D. J., Ukoumunne, O. C., Fleming, L. E., & Osborne, N. J. Prevalence, associated factors, and comorbid conditions for Meniere's disease. Ear and hearing, 2014, **35**(4), e162-e169.

Section 4

Ménière's Disease - Pathophysiology

Chapter 4

Caffeine and Meniere's Disease

Alleluia Lima Losno Ledesma,
Monique Antunes de Souza Chelminski Barreto and
Carlos Augusto Costa Pires de Oliveira

Additional information is available at the end of the chapter

http://dx.doi.org/10.5772/intechopen.69667

Abstract

Meniere's disease is characterized by recurrent vertigo, fluctuating hearing loss, and persistent tinnitus. Caffeine consumption in modern society is a widespread and culturally accepted habit; however, there is no consensus about its mechanism of action in various organs and systems, including the auditory and vestibular. The few clinical studies have shown that abstention from caffeine has little effect in patients with Meniere's disease, both in relation to vertigo, tinnitus and hearing loss.

Keywords: caffeine, vertigo, Meniere's diseases, tinnitus, vestibular disease

1. Introduction

Caffeine consumption in modern society is a widespread and culturally accepted habit and sets up the most widely consumed psychoactive substance in the world. It is found in a variety of products such as coffee, tea, chocolate, soft drinks, mate, guarana powder, slimming drugs, diuretics, stimulants, painkillers, and anti-allergics [1, 2].

The effects of caffeine have been investigated for a long time; however, there is still no consensus on the effect of this substance in the body [1]. Its action and its effect on the body are still controversial in the scientific literature. They are described as benefits the improvement of cognitive and psychomotor performance, alertness, attention span, attention, and memory; enhances visual and auditory vigilance; and decreases sleepiness and fatigue [3]. It also describes that it may cause tachycardia, increased gastric secretion, diuresis, increased levels of fatty acids in the plasma, cerebral vascular constriction, and dilation system of the other vessels of the body when in high doses [1].

INTECH
open science | open minds

© 2017 The Author(s). Licensee InTech. This chapter is distributed under the terms of the Creative Commons Attribution License (http://creativecommons.org/licenses/by/3.0), which permits unrestricted use, distribution, and reproduction in any medium, provided the original work is properly cited. (cc) BY

Meniere's disease is a clinical syndrome that affects the inner ear, and it is characterized by episodes of spontaneous vertigo, usually associated with unilateral fluctuating sensorineural hearing loss (SNHL), tinnitus, and aural fullness [4]. It is believed that there is an association between the use or caffeine abstention with complaints of vertigo and tinnitus. However, the evidence supporting this claim is conflicting and sparse [5, 6].

2. Caffeine and its effects on metabolism

Caffeine is the most consumed psychoactive substance in the world and is found in many different products such as coffee, tea, chocolate, soft drinks, mate, guarana powder, diuretics, stimulants, analgesics, and anti-allergic [1].

Caffeine (1, 3, 7-trimethylxanthine) is a stimulant of the central nervous system belonging to the group of methylxanthines [2, 7, 8]. The interaction of caffeine with the organism is difficult to research because factors such as age, presence of chronic diseases, gender, and intake of other substances such as tobacco interfere with this interaction [8].

It is believed that, with regard to pharmacokinetics, caffeine has rapid absorption, 99% absorbed within 45 minutes after its ingestion [9, 10]. It is fat-soluble, being able to overcome all biological barriers [1, 10]. The plasma concentration in humans is achieved between15 and 120 minutes after intake [11]. In humans, doses below 10 mg/kg have half-life by 2.5–4.5 hours and was not related difference in young and elderly subjects [1, 10].

Caffeine improves cognitive and psychomotor performance, alertness, ability to concentrate, attention, and memory; improves auditory and visual vigilance; and reduces sleepiness and fatigue [3]. Caffeine in high doses can cause tachycardia, increased gastric secretion, diuresis, increased levels of fatty acids in plasma, constriction in the cerebral vascular system, and expansion of other vessels of the body [1].

In otorhinolaryngology (ENT)/audiology, it has been linked to several symptoms and diseases, such as tinnitus, hydrops, dizziness, laryngopharynx acid reflux disease (LPRD), and as a risk factor for head and neck cancer [5, 6].

Caffeine mechanism of action for the production of these effects has not been fully elucidated. However, it is known that the caffeine molecule is chemically similar to other metabolically important compounds such as purines (adenine, guanine), adenosine, xanthine, and uric acid. Due to the structural similarity of caffeine molecule with adenosine, caffeine connects itself to adenosine A1 and A2A receptors, blocking them. Thus, adenosine cannot perform their inhibitory effect, which occurs through the release of several neurotransmitters, such as glutamate, acetylcholine, monoamines, and gamma-aminobutyric acid [8, 12].

Other effects such as the inhibition of phosphodiesterase (cAMP enzyme inactivating) and release of intracellular calcium are also described, however, occur only at high doses of caffeine, which cannot be achieved only with the coffee intake [8, 10]. It is suggested that the mechanisms are unrelated to the central effects of caffeine [13].

Studies suggest that caffeine also has a vasoconstrictor effect, especially when binds to A2 receptors. Functional magnetic resonance demonstrated a reduction in cerebral perfusion after caffeine intake. Nonetheless, this is the predominant effect at high doses [13].

There are over a hundred years had been reported that the abrupt discontinuation of the act of drinking coffee can cause severe headaches [12, 14]. The most common symptoms of the withdrawal of caffeine are headache, fatigue, lethargy, flu-like symptoms, and mood disorders [15]. These effects appear 12–14 hours after discontinuation of caffeine consumption and dissipate between 4 and 7 days after their occurrence [16]. The intensity of the symptoms seems to depend on the dose of caffeine that the individual usually ingest [17], although it has been reported in sporadic consumers [18]. The authors add that, despite a dose-dependent, caffeine is not effective to alleviate the symptoms caused by one's abstinence.

3. Caffeine and Meniere's disease

Meniere's disease is characterized by recurrent vertigo, fluctuating hearing loss, and persistent tinnitus [19]. The traditional treatment for Meniere's disease involves, in addition to medication and surgical procedures when indicated, a diet that restricts sodium, caffeine, and alcohol [20].

Some authors argue that the treatment of Meniere's disease is empirical and propose food restriction as an initial treatment step, not justifying the need to abstain from caffeine [21]. The recommendation of a diet free of caffeine for Meniere's disease is based on the professional's experience, without scientific evidence [22].

It was believed that sodium restriction followed the same idea of the use of diuretics, or reduced fluid retention in the inner ear. However, it was proved that the critical feature is the sodium level constant [20].

The justification for the recommendation given to Meniere's disease patients to avoid salt is the same to avoid caffeine. It is based on the theory that considers Hydrops as a cause, not symptoms of the disease. They believed that this substance causes large fluid shifts through physiologic compartments and hence result in inner ear instability [6]. Nonetheless, a cross-over study did not find significant effect of caffeine on hydratation status when body weight and urinary output were measured [23].

Using the keywords "Meniere's disease" and "caffeine," in PubMed, only one clinical study was found seeking to investigate this relationship (see **Table 1**).

Seeking to verify adherence to a diet consisting of control the sodium and caffeine, in patients with Meniere's disease, a retrospective study was conducted. The numbers of crises and the severity of symptoms decrease, as reported by the participants; however, no statistical significance was found when we analyzed only limited caffeine consumption. Fewer participants were able to restrict caffeine intake compared to reducing sodium intake. The authors suggest

Author, origin, and year of publication	Study design	Sample size	Conclusion
Luxford et al., USA, 2013 [22]	Mailed patient retrospective questionnaire and chart review	136	No statistical significance was found when analyzed only limit caffeine consumption in relation to the numbers of crisis and the severity of symptoms

Table 1. Presentation of articles: "Meniere's disease" and "caffeine".

the need for prospective controlled studies to reduce the variables found, adding up to more conclusive results [22].

Another study aiming to characterize the patients with Meniere's disease found that 30.1% use decaffeinated coffee, higher percentage than the 19% who make use of this type of coffee in the control group. The authors complete that this restriction is based on limited evidence but are extremely well publicized in the media [24].

Caffeine consumption and interruption has been related to the trigger dizziness, tinnitus, and migraine. In clinical practice, discontinuation of caffeine intake is a common recommendation for patients with these symptoms. However, some professionals report that despite well meaning this is a painful recommendation and may aggravate the discomfort reported by the patient as it can add the effects of caffeine withdrawal syndrome [5, 25].

4. Caffeine and vestibular system

Three systems (vestibular, visual, and proprioceptive) interact with each other to ensure the body balance. The vestibular system has three functions: to provide information about body position, correct body movements that deviate from its center of mass, and control eye movement to keep the visual motor while the individual or the environment is in motion [26, 27].

The posterior labyrinth is a highly sensitive organ to changes in other organs and systems, and many of these changes manifest themselves primarily with vestibular symptoms. It is related to cervical problems, cardiovascular problems, migraine, metabolic and/or hormonal changes, psychiatric disorders, neurological diseases, and the use of medications such as antibiotics, anti-inflammatories, diuretics, and psychotropic substances with labyrinthine disorders [28–31].

Investigating the vestibulocochlear findings in patients with Type 1 diabetes mellitus was found large percentage of vestibular disorders in these patients (60%). Regarding the complaints and harmful eating habits, caffeine abuse was the most prevalent of them, reported by 20% of patients [32].

The effectiveness of cessation of caffeine consumption in remission of dizziness was investigated previously. For this purpose, patients received this orientation, only being used drug treatment if symptoms persist 4 weeks after the initiation of restriction. Only 14% of participants reported some improvement in symptoms in the period in which it was only oriented diet. The authors add that patients reported improvement in general had lower consumption of caffeine in the usual diet than those who maintained their complaint after the restriction [25].

In patients with complaints of dizziness is always recommended an evaluation of the vestibular system [33]. To perform these tests, most services suspended the intake of foods high in caffeine, nonessential drugs, tobacco, and alcohol. As for the number of hours of restrictive diet, some authors suggest 72 hours suspension before the exam [27, 34, 35], some 48 hours before [36], and some even 24 hours before the test [28, 37].

Regarding the use of caffeine restriction to conduct vestibular tests, they were found only four studies in the literature. All they found weak relationship between caffeine consumption and changes in the tests, as shown the next.

In 2005, a comparative study was conducted, in which the study group and the control group were formed by the same patients in normal habits and caffeine restriction. Patients received as instruction for the first vestibular test (vectoelectronystagmography): fast 3 hours before the test, suspension of nonessential drugs and alcohol (72 hours before the test), and cigarette and products containing caffeine (24 hours before). The second test had the same guidelines except the restriction of the use of products containing caffeine. Most participants (68.4%) chose to undergo the examination with the habitual intake of caffeine. The most frequent complaints during the examination caffeine abstention were anxiety (92.3%), headache (69.3%), nausea and/or vomiting (38.5%), and more intense vertigo during the test (38.5%). As the result of the examination, no abnormality was found in the oculomotor tests and there was no statistically significant change between the responses found in the caloric test [38].

A study performed with 30 healthy young individuals aimed to investigate the influence of caffeine on vectoelectronystagmography and VEMP. For this, they performed the tests twice, once with 24-hour restriction of the use of caffeine and other after drinking a cup of coffee. The results showed that moderate caffeine consumption did not influence the test results [17].

A prospective experimental study investigated the influence of caffeine on VEMP. It was recommended, to 25 healthy young, caffeine abstinence for at least 24 hours. They were submitted to the first examination, after given caffeine capsules (420 mg) and performed the second test. There was no caffeine influence on test results [39].

A study aimed to investigate the effect of caffeine on dynamic posturography examination investigating the vestibular-spinal reflex. We investigated 30 healthy young subjects, being conducted a session where they were instructed to abstain from caffeine intake for 24 hours and another where it was offered coffee before the exam. The authors concluded that caffeine did not affect the clinical interpretation of the test in this population [40].

Table 2 summarizes the findings of clinical studies that linked caffeine and the vestibular system.

Author, origin, and year of publication	Study design	Sample size	Conclusion
Felipe et al., Brazil, 2005 [38]	Clinical with transversal cohort	19	The moderate ingestion of coffee was not shown to interfere in the results of the vestibular test
Klagenberg et al., Brazil, 2007 [32]	Cross-sectional study of a contemporary group	30	Significant vestibular system changes were found
Mikulec et al., USA, 2012 [25]	Retrospective chart review	44	Only 14% of participants reported some improvement in symptoms in the period in which it was only oriented diet
McNerney et al., USA, 2014 [17]	Prospective, placebo controlled study	30	Moderate amount of caffeine does not have a clinically significant effect on the results from caloric and cVEMP tests in young healthy adults
McNerney et al., USA, 2014 [40]	Prospective, placebo controlled study	30	The ingestion of caffeine did not produce a clinically significant effect in healthy young control participants
Sousa and Suzuki, Brazil, 2014 [39]	Prospective experimental study	25	The vestibulocollic reflex is not altered by caffeine intake

Table 2. Presentation of articles: "vestibular system" and "caffeine".

5. Caffeine and tinnitus

Tinnitus is a sound that is perceived in the absence of an external acoustic stimulus. The pathophysiology of this symptom has not been fully elucidated, in part related to the subjective nature of this condition, associated with emotional and psychological factors accompanying its occurrence [41, 42].

A retrospective study was conducted aiming to investigate the correlation of the presence of habits and symptoms with the annoyance of tinnitus. Dizziness, neck pain, headache, and caffeine abuse are prevalent complaints in patients with tinnitus. However, there was no correlation among the degree of annoyance of tinnitus with hearing loss, age, gender, presence of dizziness, neck pain, headache, changes of the temporomandibular joint, and the use of caffeine or excessive intake of carbohydrates [43].

It is observed in clinical practice, including being reported in the literature, the recommendation of discontinuation of caffeine as additional treatment for tinnitus. This recommendation is based on the theoretical deduction that if caffeine has stimulating action on the central nervous system, it can play a role in the excitability of the auditory pathways and, therefore, can modify some clinical aspects of tinnitus [13].

There was not, however, scientific evidence for this recommendation. Recently, the search for scientific evidence of this recommendation was prospectively investigated in three studies presented in **Table 3**. In none of them significant improvement in annoyance was observed due to tinnitus only with the reduction of caffeine consumption.

A phase 2, pseudo-randomized, double-blind, placebo-controlled cross-over trial was conducted to test the causal relationship between caffeine consumption and tinnitus severity. Specific questionnaires were applied to investigate the annoyance due to tinnitus and visual analogue scale at base line and on days 1, 15, and 30. The groups, study, and placebo were matched. Authors concluded that caffeine content had no effect on tinnitus severity and increase headaches and nausea [5].

Using the answers from the Nurses' Health Study II, a series of questionnaires applied in women aged 25–42 years, the authors sought to examine the association between caffeine intake and the risk of incident tinnitus. After analyzing the data, the study concluded that after adjusting age and potential confounders there was a significant inverse association between caffeine intake and the incidence of tinnitus [44].

Seeking to assess whether tinnitus patients can obtain some benefit from the reduction of caffeine intake, 26 patients with tinnitus were advised to reduce caffeine consumption by 50% of regular consumption. Audiometry being carried out and applied the tinnitus handicap inventory (THI) and visual analogic scale (VAS) before and after reduction consumption. The authors argue that despite the statistical significance of data found, clinical improvement was small. Adds that the greater the amount of caffeine consumed, the greater the impact caused by the reduction of intake, which could be responsible for a possible worsening of tinnitus, related to caffeine withdrawal. The fact indicates that there is no justification for the universal restriction of caffeine intake as a treatment for all patients with tinnitus; however, some groups are more likely to improve [13].

Author, origin and year of publication	Study design	Sample size	Conclusion
Claire et al., UK, 2010 [5]	A phase 2, pseudo-randomized, double-blind, placebo-controlled cross-over trial	66	Caffeine content had no effect on tinnitus severity and increase headaches and nausea
Glicksman et al., USA, 2014 [44]	Longitudinal and prospective study	5289	Higher caffeine intake was associated with a lower risk of incident tinnitus in women
Figueiredo et al., Brazil, 2014 [13]	Contemporary longitudinal cohort study	26	There is no justification for the universal restriction of caffeine intake as a treatment for all patients with tinnitus

Table 3. Presentation of articles: "tinnitus" and "caffeine".

6. Caffeine and auditory system

A larger number of studies have been found attempting to investigate the effects of caffeine in the auditory system. It is believed that caffeine affected the peripheral and central auditory pathways [45]. As the inner ear is the site of lesion for this clinical syndrome, we direct our efforts in presenting the effects of caffeine on the peripheral auditory system [46].

Regard to the effects of caffeine on the peripheral auditory system, it was demonstrated that caffeine induced shortening of outer hair cells, increasing the excitability of the peripheral auditory pathways [47]. The mechanism of action that provides this shortening has not been fully elucidated [13]. It was suggested that caffeine induced contraction by activating the ryanodine receptor, by potassium channel blockage or by creating osmotic imbalance across the cell membrane [47–49].

No clinical studies in humans to investigate the relationship of caffeine to the peripheral auditory system were found.

7. Conclusion

Caffeine despite being widely consumed has no mechanism of action fully elucidated. The vestibular and auditory systems may be influenced by substances that alter the homeostasis of the organism. Thus, while the interaction of caffeine with cochlea and the posterior labyrinth is not better elucidated, the diet recommendations for evaluation and therapy of patients with vertigo and tinnitus remain based on clinical experience. It will be finally necessary more studies to elucidate these questions aiding in driving the most effective treatment for the patient with Meniere's disease.

Author details

Alleluia Lima Losno Ledesma*, Monique Antunes de Souza Chelminski Barreto and Carlos Augusto Costa Pires de Oliveira

*Address all correspondence to: luafono@yahoo.com.br

University of Brasília, Brazil

References

[1] Chou T. Wake up and smell the coffee –.Caffeine, coffee and the medical consequences. Western Journal Medicine. 1992;**157**(5):544-553

[2] Camargo MCR, Toledo MCF. Teor de cafeína em cafés brasileiros. Journal of Food Science and Technology. 1998;**18**(4):421-424. DOI: 10.1590/S0101-20611998000400012

[3] Lima DR. O Café pode ser bom para a saúde. In: Simpósio de pesquisa dos cafés do Brasil. Brasília: Embrapa; 2002. pp. 195-229. Available at: http://www.sbicafe.ufv.br/handle/123456789/538

[4] Frejo L, Giegling I, Teggi R, Lopez-Escamez JA, Rujescu D. Genetics of vestibular disorders: Pathophysiological insights. Journal of Neurology. 2016;**263**(1):45-53. DOI: 10.1007/s00415-015-7988-9

[5] Claire LS, Stothart G, Mckenna L, Rogers PJ. Caffeine abstinence: An ineffective and potentially distressing tinnitus therapy. International Journal of Audiology. 2010;**49**(1):24-29. DOI: 10.3109/14992020903160884

[6] Trindade A, Robinson T, Phillips JS. The role of caffeine in otorhinolaryngology: Guilty as charged? European Archives of Oto-Rhino-Laryngology. 2014;**271**(8):2097-2102. DOI: 10.1007/s00405-013-2648-0

[7] Mycek MJ, Harvey RA, Champe PC. Estimulantes do SNC. In: Finkel R, editor. Farmacologia ilustrada. Porto Alegre: ArTmed; 1998. pp. 462-478

[8] Alves RC, Casal S, Oliveira B. Health benefits of coffee: Myth or reality? Química Nova. 2009;**32**(8):2169-2180. DOI: 10.1590/S0100-40422009000800031

[9] Denaro CP, Brown CR, Jacob P, Benowitz NL. Effects of caffeine with repeated dosing. European Journal of Clinical Pharmacology.1991;**40**(3):273-278

[10] Fredholm BB, Bättig K, Holmén J, Nehlig A, Zvartau E. Actions of caffeine in the brain with special reference to factors that contribute to its widespread use. Pharmacological Review. 1999;**51**(1):83-133

[11] Bonati M, Latini R, Galletti F, Young JF, Tognoni G, Garattini S. Caffeine disposition after oral doses. Clinical Pharmacology & Therapeutics. 1982;**32**(1):98-106

[12] James JE. Caffeine & Health. Londres: Academic Press; 1991. p. 432

[13] Figueiredo RR, Rates MJA, Azevedo AA, Moreira RKP, Penido NO. Effects of the reduction of caffeine consumption on tinnitus perception. Brazilian Journal of Otorhinolaryngology. 2014;**80**(5):416-421

[14] Siqueira TV. A cultura do café: 1961-2005. Rio de Janeiro: BNDES Setorial; 2005

[15] Silverman K, Evans SM, Strain EC, Griffiths RR. Withdrawal syndrome after the double-blind cessation of caffeine consumption. The New England Journal of Medicine. 1992;**327**:1109-1114. DOI: 10.1056/NEJM199210153271601

[16] Evans SM, Griffiths RR. Caffeine withdrawal: A parametric analysis of caffeine dosing conditions. The Journal of Pharmacology and Experimental Therapeutics. 1999;**289**:285-294

[17] McNerney K, Coad Ml, Burkard R. The influence of caffeine on calorics and cervical vestibular evoked myogenic potentials (cVEMPs). Journal of the American Academy of Audiology. 2014;**25**:261-267. DOI: 10.3766/jaaa.25.3.5

[18] Strain EC, Griffths RR. Caffeine dependence: Fact or fiction? Journal of the Royal Society of Medicine. 1995;**88**(8):437-440

[19] Kitahara T, Okamoto H, Fukushima M, Sakagami M, Ito T, Yamashita A, Ota I, Yamanaka T. A two-year randomized trial of interventions to decrease stress hormone vasopressin production in patients with Meniere's disease – A pilot study. PLoS ONE. 2016;**11**(6):e0158309. DOI: 10.1371/journal.pone.0158309

[20] Rauch SD. Clinical hints and precipitating factors in patients suffering from Meniere's disease. Otolaryngologic Clinics of North America. 2010;**43**(5):1011-1017. DOI: http://dx.doi.org/10.1016/j.otc.2010.05.003

[21] Knox GW, McPherson A. Ménière's disease: Differential diagnosis and treatment. American Family Physician. 1997;**55**(4):1185-1190

[22] Luxford E, Berliner KI, Lee J, Luxford WM. Dietary modification as adjunct treatment in Ménière's disease: Patient willingness and ability to comply. Otology and Neurotology. 2013;**34**(8):1438-1443. DOI: http://dx.doi.org/10.1097/MAO.0b013e3182942261

[23] Grandjean AC, Reimers KJ, Bannick KE, Haven MC. The effect of caffeinated, non-caffeinated, caloric and non-caloric beverages on hydration. The Journal of the American College of Nutrition. 2000;**19**:591-600

[24] Tyrrell JS, Whinney DJD, Ukoumunne OC, Fleming LE, Osborne NJ. Prevalence, associated factors, and comorbid conditions for Ménière's disease. Ear and Hearing. 2014;**35**(4):e162-e169. DOI: 10.1097/AUD.0000000000000041

[25] Mikulec AA, Faraji FF, Kinsella LJ. Evaluation of the efficacy of caffeine cessation, nortriptyline, and topiramate therapy in vestibular migraine and complex dizziness of unknown etiology. American Journal of Otolaryngology. 2012;**33**(1):121-127. DOI: http://dx.doi.org/10.1016/j.amjoto.2011.04.010

[26] Shepard NT, Telian SA. Avaliação do funcionamento do sistema vestibular. In: Katz J, editor. Tratado de Audiologia Clínica. 4th ed. São Paulo: Manole; 1999. pp. 421-443

[27] Flores MR, Franco ES. Computerized vectoelectronystamography: Pós nystagmus testing by caloric air stimulation in individuals without complaints. International Archives of Otorhinolaryngology. 2003;**7**(4):252-256

[28] Paulino CA, Prezotto AO, Calixto RF. Association between stress, depression and dizziness: A brief review. Revista Equilíbrio Corporal e Saúde (RECES). 2009;**1**(1):33-45. DOI: 10.17921/2176-9524.2009v1n1p%25p

[29] Cal R, Bahmad Jr, F. Migraine associated with auditory-vestibular dysfunction. Brazilian Journal of Otorhinolaryngology. 2008;**74**(4):606-612. DOI: 10.1590/S0034-72992008000400020

[30] Bittar RSM, Bottino MA, Simoceli L, Venosa AR. Vestibular impairment secondary to glucose metabolic disorders: Reality or myth? Brazilian Journal of Otorhinolaryngology. 2004;**70**(6):800-805. DOI: 10.1590/S0034-72992004000600016

[31] Tiensoli LO, Couto ER, Mitre EI. Vertigo or dizziness associated factors in individuals with normal vestibular function test. Revista CEFAC. 2004;**6**(1):94-100

[32] Klagenberg KF, Zeigelboim BS, Jurkiewicz AL, Martins-Basseto J. Vestibulocochlear manifestations in patients with type I diabetes mellitus. Brazilian Journal of Otorhinolaryngology. 2007;**73**(3):353-358

[33] Mor R, Fragoso M, Taguchi CK, Figueiredo JFFR. Vestibulometria na prática Fonoaudiológica. São Paulo: Pulso; 2012

[34] Mariotto LDF, Alvarenga KF, Filho OAC. Avaliação vestibular na perda auditiva sensórioneural unilateral: Estudo vesto-eletronistagmográfico. Disturbios da Comunicação. 2006;**18**(1):27-38

[35] Fukunaga JY, Ganança CF, Perrella ACM, Makibara RR, Quitschal RM, et al. Ice air caloric test in normal subjects. Acta Otolaryngol. 2009;**27**(1):27-31

[36] Koga KA, Resende BD, Mor R. Study of giddinness/vertigo related to head position changes and vestibular disorders associated to computerized vectoelectronystagmography. Revista. CEFAC. 2004;**6**(2):197-202

[37] Ruwer SL, Rossi AG, Simon LF (2005) Balance in the elderly. Brazilian Journal of Otorhinolaryngology. 2005;**71**(3):298-303. DOI: 10.1016/S1808-8694(15)31326-4

[38] Felipe L, Simões LC, Gonçalves DU, Mancini PC. Evaluation of the caffeine effect in the vestibular test. Brazilian Journal of Otorhinolaryngology. 2005;**71**(6):758-762

[39] Sousa AMA, Suzuki FA. Effect of caffeine on cervical vestibular-evoked myogenic potential in healthy individuals. Brazilian Journal of Otorhinolaryngology. 2014;**80**(3):26-30. http://dx.doi.org/10.1016/j.bjorl.2014.02.004

[40] McNerney K, Coad Ml, Burkard R. The influence of caffeine on the sensory organization test. Journal of the American Academy of Audiology. 2014;**25**:521-528. DOI: 10.3766/jaaa.25.6.2

[41] Jastreboff PJ, Hazell JW. A neurophysiological approach to tinnitus: Clinical implications. British Journal of Audiology. 1993;**27**:7-17. DOI: 10.3109/03005369309077884

[42] Alsalman OA, Tucker D, Vanneste S. Salivary Stress-Related responses in tinnitus: A preliminary study in young male subjects with tinnitus. Frontiers in Neuroscience. 2016;**20**(10):338. DOI: 10.3389/fnins.2016.00338.

[43] Valente JPP, Pinheiro LAM, Carvalho GM, Guimarães AC, Mezzalira R, Stoler G, Paschoal JR, et al. Evaluation of factors related to the tinnitus disturbance. International Tinnitus Journal. 2012;**17**(1):21-25

[44] Glicksman JT, Curhan SG, Curhan GC. A prospective study of caffeine intake and risk of incident tinnitus. American Journal of Medicine. 2014;**127**(8):739-743. DOI: 10.1016/j.amjmed.2014.02.033.

[45] Dixit A, Vaney N, Tandon OP. Effect of caffeine on central auditory pathways: An evoked potential study. Hearing Research. 2006;**220**(1-2):61-66. DOI:10.1016/j.heares.2006.06.017

[46] Gürkov R, Pyykö I, Zou J, Kentala E. What is Menière's disease? A contemporary re-evaluation of endolymphatic hydrops. Journal of Neurology. 2016;**263**(Suppl 1):71-81. DOI: 10.1007/s00415-015-7930-1

[47] Slepecky S, Ulfendahl M, Flock A. Effects of caffeine and tetracaine on outer hair cells shortening suggest intracellular calcium involvement. Hearing Research. 1988;**32**:11-22

[48] Yamamoto T, Kakehata S, Yamada T, Saito T, Saito H, Akaike N. Caffeine rapidly decreases potassium conductance of dissociated outer hair cells of guinea pig cochlea. Brain Research. 1995;**677**:89-96

[49] Skellett RA, Crist JR, Fallon M, Bobbin RP. Caffeine-induced shortening of isolated outer hair cells: an osmotic mechanism of action. Hearing Research. 1995;**87**:41-48

Chapter 5

Pathophysiology of Meniere's Disease

Shazia Mirza and Sankalp Gokhale

Additional information is available at the end of the chapter

http://dx.doi.org/10.5772/66388

Abstract

Meniere's disease, with its characteristic symptom triad of vertigo, balance and hearing disorders has yet to have its pathophysiology outlined conclusively. Any theory must elucidate all aspects of the natural progression, including vestibular and auditory symptoms. While the central dogma revolves around endolymphatic hydrops, this theory is not without flaws, such as its inability to explain all the physiological changes seen in patients, or the often absence of symptoms. While several degenerative changes are observed in temporal bone histopathology, they do not necessarily explain the sequence of events in the development and progress of the disease. This chapter explores the pathophysiology of the disease, focusing on the hydrops theory, while presenting evidence for and against it. Various changes in the inner ear physiology such as pressure changes, ionic disequilibrium, endocochlear potentials; in human and animal models are described. Alternative explanations for symptoms are discussed. This chapter touches briefly upon etiology associated with Meniere's (and hydrops), and aims to assist a deeper understanding of the relationship of the process to clinical and experimental findings. A clear understanding of the process guides not only the clinical management to improve quality of life but also the direction of future research endeavors.

Keywords: Meniere's disease, pathophysiology, etiology, mechanism, endolymphatic hydrops, deafness, vertigo

1. Introduction

Meniere's disease, with a symptom triad of vertigo, balance and hearing disorders, was reported as a disease of the inner ear by Prosper Meniere as far back as 1861 [1] and has yet to have its pathophysiology defined conclusively. Since a central theory of the pathophysiology involves endolymphatic hydrops, it is worthwhile be familiar with the terms.

INTECH
open science | open minds

© 2017 The Author(s). Licensee InTech. This chapter is distributed under the terms of the Creative Commons Attribution License (http://creativecommons.org/licenses/by/3.0), which permits unrestricted use, distribution, and reproduction in any medium, provided the original work is properly cited.

Endolymph is the potassium-rich fluid in the membranous labyrinth, produced by the stria vascularis (cells in the scala media) of the cochlear labyrinth along with some contribution from the dark vestibular cells and planum semilunatum. There is a slow longitudinal flow and a fast radial flow of endolymph, also influenced by osmotic and hydrostatic forces. Endolymphatic hydrops refers to the over-accumulation of endolymph, pressing upon the perilymphatic space resulting in the characteristic symptom triad. The exact mechanism of this hydrops is unknown and can range from over-production, decreased absorption, to mechanical obstruction. If the cause of the distension or hydrops is unknown, the syndrome can be termed Meniere's disease (MD); conversely, if the cause is known, it is termed secondary endolymphatic blockage. The chapter intends to outline mechanisms for the hydrops; however, this theory is plagued with controversy as shown in a study of cadaveric temporal bone specimens wherein 100% of the diagnosed MD patients had evidence of hydrops, contrasted by findings of hydrops in 51/79 patients without an MD diagnosis, highlighting gaps in this theory [2].

2. Historical journey in pathophysiology

Prosper Meniere in 1861 observed the constellation of symptoms (such as tinnitus, hearing loss, falls, vertigo, nausea and syncope), when he postulated that the ear was the site of the disorder in contrast to the popular theory of apoplectiform cerebral congestion [1]. Building upon Flourens' experiments on pigeons, he further refined the site of the lesion to be the semicircular canals. In 1938, two independent studies by Yamakawa (in Japan) and Hallpike and Cairns (In England) described the hydrops as a pathological finding of the labyrinth; these anatomical findings were confirmed by various investigators through the decade to come [2].

3. Pathophysiology

MD is characterized during its active phase with the characteristic symptom triad, of episodic vertigo and tinnitus with fluctuations in hearing, followed by a symptom-free period, ultimately resulting in a more permanent dysfunction of the above symptoms. Any theory attempting to explain the pathophysiology of MD has to account for processes that result in a reversible dysfunction of both the cochlea and vestibule, with long-term chronic deficits. Examples of reversible causes include noise, toxins such as salicylates, viral infections and immune-mediated mechanisms, most of which do not show morphological changes unless they turn permanent.

This suggests a possibility of a final common pathway in a variety of conditions that could all result in fluctuating cochlear and vestibular dysfunction. The exact mechanisms are not clearly elucidated, with noise-related damage being a notable exception. In all cases, a persistence of the metabolic dysfunction results in permanence. Hence, it may be inferred that MD is modeled on the pathophysiology of disorders wherein abnormalities of metabolic dysfunction result in a permanent vestibulocochlear dysfunction.

http://dx.doi.org/10.5772/66388

The problem in MD is thought to be malabsorption of endolymph, mainly in the duct or sac. This outflow dysfunction is usually a slow process, the inciting etiological event having occurred possibly years earlier.

4. Central theory of Meniere's disease

In simple terms, the central hypothesis of Meniere's disease pathophysiology is endolymphatic hydrops, due to a varied etiology (auto-immune, infectious, endocrine, allergic, vascular, autonomic, dietary, genetic, idiopathic, etc.) and is responsible for the symptoms of MD.

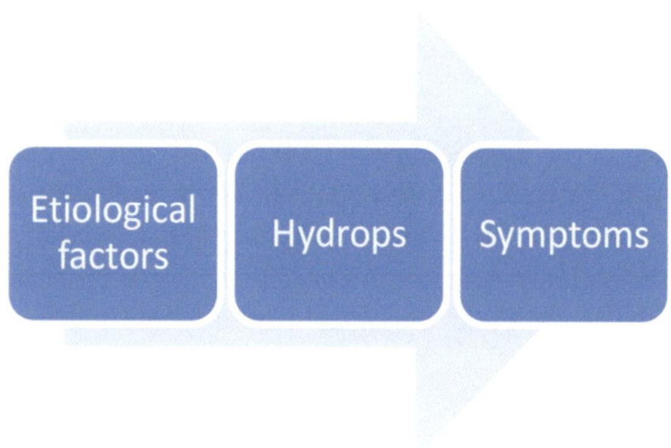

A discussion on the central theory necessarily focuses on the events leading up to the hydrops and the physiological consequences of the hydrops. Endolymphatic hydrops is the only consistently found anatomical abnormality in MD, with volume increases up to 200% in patients of MD versus health patients [3]. This correlation, however, does not imply causality, for if hydrops was causative then not only would every patient with Meniere's disease have hydrops but also the reverse; every case of hydrops would have symptoms of Meniere's disease, a statement we know does not stand true [2].

The theory regards that excess endolymph is due to overproduction or reduced resorption, either idiopathic or due to various etiologies, most likely being obstruction at the level of the duct or sac, which results in EH. The acuteness of attacks can be explained by the increased pressures within the scala media which result in a rupture of the membranous labyrinth. These ruptures are expected to occur frequently in MD and have been found in all parts of the inner ear in MD patients along with healed scars. This possibly explains the sudden attacks and fluctuation of symptoms. The Schuknecht theory is prominent for highlighting the ionic changes; ruptures of the membranous labyrinth cause a mixing of potassium-rich endolymph into the perilymph. This potassium is excitotoxic when exposed to CN VIII and hair cells as it causes depolarization of the nerve cells and subsequent inactivation. This results in decreased cochlear and vestibular function and symptoms of a Meniere's attack. When the ruptured membrane heals, symptoms subside [4].

While other pathological findings in hydrops include membrane ruptures, periductal sclerosis, damage to hair cells and spiral ganglion cells, studies also highlight other differences observed such as abnormal glycoprotein metabolism in the endolymphatic sac. And while fibrosis around the sac need not be present in each case of MD, the widespread glycoprotein imbalance could be of value in explaining EH formation through osmotic effect affecting inner ear homeostasis [5].

Hydrops has been experimentally found to be large enough to extend into the semicircular canal and thus disrupt the crista ampullaris, responsible for vertigo. The mechanical disruption of wave conduction by the hydrops is linked to the cochlear dysfunction.

Obstruction sites other than the duct and sac (secondary sites) such as in the ductus reunions may be responsible for the predominance of cochlear symptoms. Other involved sites (such as overactive vestibular cells and planum semilunatum) may result in excess production and mainly vestibular symptoms [6].

A combination of the mechanical and chemical factors is likely to be in play in the pathophysiology of MD. Since most of the theories on MD are derived from the study of temporal bone anatomy, the pathophysiology of MD has been inferred from the observed pathology. This is not always an ideal correlation as several insults, such as noise, can alter cochlear function without altering structure. Hence, one has to exercise caution while inferring the clinical condition of Meniere's disease from the pathological condition of hydrops.

4.1. Role played by the central theory

The central theory has not only dominated the pathophysiological dogma of MD but also influenced the design of various tests such as glycerol test or potential ratios (AP/SP; explained later) used to diagnose the "hydrops" and by extension MD. Most medical and surgical therapies in practice and in research are aimed at reducing the "hydrops." Animal models are designed to recreate the "hydrops" as a model for MD. Most research is focused on discovering various etiologies or mechanisms of hydrops.

4.2. Etiology of the hydrops

Specific causes of hydrops include infectious (viruses and syphilis), allergic, genetic, trauma, autoimmune, otoconia or otoliths and low cerebrospinal fluid (CSF) pressures.

Viruses: Studies testing the endolymphatic sac of MD patients show the presence of viral DNA notably Varicella-Zoster virus (VZV), Epstein-Barr virus, cytomegalovirus and conflictingly absence of herpes simples viruses 1 and 2 [7] or its presence in the vestibular ganglion [8], with inactive serum titers during attacks, leading to a statistically based theory of latent inactive viral infections related to MD, with possible early VZV infection in childhood affecting the endolymphatic sac later in life. However, antiviral medications have no role in the treatment of MD.

Syphilis: Congenital or acquired syphilis was found to be the cause of MD in 6% of all cases, with pathogenesis of endolymphatic hydrops and osteitis of the capsule believed to cause the symptoms. This entity responds to steroid administration [9].

Hereditary: 34% of patients report a family history of hearing loss or recurrent vertigo, with 8.4% of patients having a relative with diagnosed definite MD. While genetic heterogeneity has been observed, most families had an autosomal-dominant inheritance pattern with anticipation. No clinical differences were found between sporadic and familial MD, except for an expected earlier onset in familial cases [10]. Studies have discovered two heterozygous single-nucleotide variants in FAM136A and DTNA genes, both from a Spanish family with three affected cases in consecutive generations, suggestive of autosomal-dominant inheritance [11] with various other gene mutations being explored in different familial groups.

Allergy: Studies found an inhalant allergy in 41.6% and a food allergy in 40.3% of patients with MD in comparison with rates of 27.6% and 17.4% in their control population [6]. The theory involves antigen exposure leading to a sudden influx of fluid into the endolymphatic sac (which is immunologically active), resulting in a rupture of Reissner's membrane. The resulting influx of potassium and its excitotoxicity causes the symptoms. Other theories involve deposition of circulating immune complex leading to inflammation. Patients on allergic immunotherapy have shown better control of their vertigo symptoms [6].

Autoimmunity: Immune stimulation of the endolymphatic sac may cause hydrops by disturbing its fluid regulatory function. This immune involvement is possibly type 2 (tissue antigen-antibody-related) or type 3 (circulating immune complex-related). A higher (30–50%) percentage of MD patients have circulating antigen-antibody complexes) compared to normal people; however, the detection of antibodies to vestibular antigens was lower (20%) and more variable. The deposition of the immune complexes possibly results in increased vascular permeability and hence an imbalance in the fluid electrolyte concentration [6]. Various cytokines such as interleukin-1alpha, tumor necrosis factor alpha, NF kappaB P65 and P50 have been found to be produced in cochlear cells such as type 1 fibrocytes and root cells of spiral ligament, demonstrating that local or systemic production of inflammatory ligands may play a role in cochlear dysfunction [12].

Otoconia: Studies using three-dimensional (3D) computerized tomography (CT) imaging in patients show that hydrops in MD patients might be caused by obstruction of the duct reunions by loose otoconia in the saccule [13].

Otitis media: Otitis media has been linked to the development of MD either later on in life (in childhood exposures, with vertiginous symptoms predominating) or concurrently with fluctuating hearing loss being the dominant presentation. The postulated pathophysiology involves the development of hydrops linked to labyrinthitis and or otitis media due to the under-development of the duct and sac due to the associated inflammatory sequelae in the mastoid [14]. Another possibility is the spread of infectious or inflammatory products into the perilymphatic space, which may disrupt the electrolyte homeostasis and osmotic pressures thus resulting in hydrops [6].

Trauma: Physical or acoustic trauma has been linked to MD through the dysfunction of cells involved in endolymphatic homeostasis or the traumatic displacement of cellular debris and otoconia which could physically or chemically result in hydrops [6]; studies in veterans with such trauma, however, do not provide adequate backing to this theory [15]. The bilaterality of MD cannot be explained in cases of unilateral trauma.

Otosclerosis: Patients with otosclerosis have been found to have symptoms of MD due to the otosclerosis enveloping the aqueduct or invading the endosteum, resulting in changes in the flow and chemical composition of endolymph and perilymph [16].

Low cerebrospinal fluid pressures: Connections between the inner ear and CSF allow pressure changes to be transmitted, notably, a drop in CSF pressures such as postoperatively, leading to decreased perilymphatic pressures and a corresponding relative endolymphatic hydrops [17].

Other mediators: nitric oxide and vasopressin: Overexpression of the inducible nitric oxide synthase enzyme results in morphological (hair cell loss) and functional changes (endocochlear threshold and potential shifts) and stria vascularis toxicity, implicated in the development of MD, along with other free radicals [18]. Vasopressin levels have been shown to increase before and after a vertigo attack in MD patients, in humans and experimental models possibly contributing to the development of hydrops [19].

5. Physiology in Meniere's disease

The pathophysiology of Meniere's disease is tied to the physiology of the hydrops, which can be induced in experimental models by obliteration or blockage of the duct and/or sac in animals at a success rate approaching 100% in guinea pigs but with more variability in other species. The experimental animal models remain deficient, with no acute attacks of MD and lack of reported vestibular dysfunction despite severe hydrops, cautioning against direct equivalence from animal to human theories. This induced hydrops, despite being an incomplete model, is used to study the effects on the labyrinthine and cochlear physiology such as electrolyte homeostasis in the fluids and membranes, pressures and potentials.

6. Ionic homeostasis and hydrops

Despite logistical and technical difficulties in obtaining tissues and fluid (as composition is usually disturbed during surgical procedures), some human and animal studies show a change in the sodium-potassium levels of the cochlear and vestibular endolymphatic fluids in MD and experimental hydrops, respectively [20]. In addition to the theory of ruptures causing spillage of potassium ions into the perilymph, another possible explanation for the ionic and fluid imbalances in hydrops was postulated to be the Na, K-ATPase enzymes found in the cochlear lateral wall. However immunohistochemical studies of human temporal bones did not show statistically significant differences in hydropic ears consistent with the normal functioning of the stria vascularis in patients with MD [21]. Possible theories diverging from the traditional disruption of Guild's principle of longitudinal endolymphatic flow include ionic disequilibrium being responsible for the hydrops. Cellular changes in Reissner's membrane are postulated to cause disruption of the endolymphatic flow and thus lead to ionic imbalance, a possible mechanism of hearing loss in endolymphatic hydrops [22].

7. Pressure changes and hydrops

Experimental models studying the effect of postural changes on endo- and perilymphatic space fluid pressures show a marked change in the hydropic versus control animals [23]. There is possibly an adaptation of the vestibular system to the increased endolymphatic pressures, given that the time period for the development of hydrops is over months. This adaptation is unlikely to remain in effect with changes in posture. This uncompensated disequilibrium of fluid pressures may be responsible for the vestibular dysfunction.

A second mechanism to consider is that an increase in pressures produced in the hydropic ear during postural changes compresses the microvasculature on the wall of the labyrinth, resulting in ischemia of the inner ear [24].

The cerebrospinal fluid pressure dictates the inner ear hydrostatic pressure through the cochlear aqueduct. Studies measuring the positional changes of intracranial CSF pressure and its corresponding effects on the perilymphatic pressures showed insignificant differences between MD affected and control ears [25]. Animal models measuring endo- and perilymphatic space fluid pressures before and after induced hydrops show no significance in pressure between the scala media and the scala tympani in either control or hydropic ears [26], with similar findings in humans, thus precluding the use of MMS-10 tympanic displacement analyzer (Marchbanks' test) in a diagnostic capacity [27].

8. Endocochlear potential and hydrops

Experimental models report a decrease in the endocochlear potential (EP) developing after inducing hydrops [26]. Measurements of the evoked responses of the cochlea such as cochlear microphonic potential (CM) show decreased maximum output and threshold levels. Auditory brainstem responses also show progressive deficits. Electrophysiological tests such as electrocochleography (ECoG) are commonly used in the diagnosis of MD which includes both the compound action potential (CAP) and the summating potential (SP). The CAP is the summation of responses from the auditory nerve which would be reduced in patients with hearing loss. The SP is the summation of responses from the hair cells. Since hydrops would push the basilar membrane closer toward the scala tympani, in the absence of hair cell damage or loss (seen in the early stages of the disease), this effect of hydrops would increase the SP. While the absolute values of these two components may differ, they do covary and hence the ratio between the two is often used in MD diagnosis.

Studies show that while rupture of the membranous labyrinth in hydrops was believed to be responsible for the inner ear dysfunction (through large volume injections into the endolymphatic sac), the pattern of pressure changes in conjunction with techniques examining temporal bones via a micro-CT and functional electrographic recordings shows that they are not solely responsible for the acute ear dysfunction, rather the hydrops is a continuing, prolonged process with Non-rupture mechanisms in play, which can be correlated clinically with MD too [28].

9. The role of CNS in MD

The CNS modulates functions of the inner ear by several mechanisms, which may have a bearing on the pathophysiology of MD. Alterations in autonomic activity may modulate vascular tone which could set off an acute attack with longer term effects resulting in a chronic damage. Since cochlear fine tuning is compromised in MD, it is likely that efferent pathways are likely to be involved in acute attacks. The role of the neuroendocrine system causing metabolic dysfunction is yet to be elucidated.

10. Physiology of clinical symptoms and hydrops

10.1. Fluctuating hearing loss and episodic vertigo

As outlined earlier, a possible explanation for the fluctuating hearing loss and episodic vertigo seen in MD patients is brief, acute rises in pressures resulting in membranous ruptures, resulting in cochleovestibular dysfunction due to ionic disequilibrium (potassium excitotoxicity). Healing of these ruptures sets the stage for symptom resolution. The correlation of electron microscopic damage visualized in animal models of hydrops, such as hair cell loss, neuronal damage and spiral ganglion cell and ligament damage, is purported to be responsible for the hearing deficits.

A physiological basis of the Hennebert sign (vertigo occurring when static pressure is applied to the ear) is the presence of vestibular fibrosis (part of the pathological manifestations of the disease which may form band-like connections between the footplate of the stapes and the utricular macula [29].

10.2. Aural fullness

Patients often complain of aural fullness (a blocked or full sensation) which, while colloquially has been attributed to the hydropic swelling, has no scientific basis due to the lack of inner ear receptors to relay this information to the brain and the improbability that a minute increase in endolymphatic volume would be adequate to stretch the round window to results in this fullness sensation. A possible explanation could be the childhood association of a common middle ear disease (otitis media) with its prominent sensation of fullness with the low-frequency hearing loss which accompanies middle ear conductive pathologies. In essence, the low-frequency hearing loss experienced by the patient is accompanied by fullness as a learned association.

10.3. Recruitment

Loudness intolerance or recruitment also seen in MD patients is due to the loss of the outer hair cell function which serves to fine-tune or evoke region-specific responses of the basilar membrane to varying frequencies. As a result, larger regions of the membrane and hence a larger population of neurons are excited for a stimulus which is usually interpreted as increased signal intensity. Altered perception of pitch, a symptom of MD, is similarly explained by the abnormal recruitment of neurons. The brain thus perceives different signals from the "normal" and the "affected" ear for a given sound, resulting in the perception of two sounds. This unusual symptom is notable in MD due to the asymmetry of the disease process.

10.4. Tinnitus

A possible explanation for the tinnitus could be related to a similar broad tuning of the cochlear membrane. A reduced functioning of the receptors and nerves at the cochlear apex may allow the CNS to interpret the boundary zone between the active cochlea and the inactive apex as tinnitus. Another mechanism could involve channels getting inputs from the inactive area of the nerve fibers, which would optimize their gain, leading to amplification of internal signals thus resulting in tinnitus.

10.5. Chronic symptoms

Irreversibility of symptoms and chronic deterioration in hearing are explained by the permanent morphological changes such as distortions in the ampulla walls, utricular macula and atrophy of the cristae. Such distensions of the lateral ampulla have been shown to be associated with impaired vestibular function tests [30]. While light microscopy may not always show obvious pathology, electron microscopy showing degeneration of unmyelinated axons may explain the symptoms such as loss of speech discrimination despite intact hair cells and spiral ganglion cells [31].

11. The evidence-based findings between hydrops and symptoms

Hyperosmolar agents and diuretics, such as glycerol and furosemide, respectively, have been used since several decades in the evaluation of patients with suspected hydrops. Several studies show that the hydrops is temporarily relieved by their mechanism of action [32–34], resulting in an improvement of hearing and or vestibular symptoms in some case, thus strengthening the case for hydrops being responsible for MD symptoms.

The results of electrocochleographic observations in MD patients also support a temporal correlation. This increase of the SP in patients with early MD, along with studies showing a positive temporal correlation of enhanced SP and symptom reporting and finally a decrease of the SP with the use of hyperosmolar agents [35], all strengthen the premise of hydrops being responsible for symptom constellation.

To explain the lack of symptoms in animal models of EH and as an alternative to the argument that hydrops cannot occur rapidly enough to cause an acute attack of symptoms, it was postulated that acute attacks of MD can be attributed to the biochemical effects of endolymphatic ruptures (not traditionally seen in animal models) specifically of Reissner's membrane. However, human temporal bone studies also do not consistently reveal theses ruptures or they have been attributed to postmortem-processing artifacts, strengthening the theory that the pressure effects along with biochemical effects act in concert. With regard to the theory that ruptures are responsible for the acute attacks, studies have questioned the likelihood of a rupture in one anatomical area impacting the function of other areas, or the likelihood of simultaneous rupture of both the cochlear duct and saccule (not supported by histology findings) affecting cochlear and vestibular functions [36]. It is also logical extension of theory to expect relief of symptoms after rupture, as relief of the pressure should alleviate symptoms.

Vestibular symptoms such as nystagmus were induced in animal models with an injection of artificial endolymph into the perilymphatic space, presumed to represent the actual events in play during an attack of episodic vertigo [37].

Imaging studies in vivo using gadolinium-contrasted magnetic resonance imaging (MRI) demonstrated that in MD, different areas affected by the EH (vestibular vs. cochlear) were correlated to different symptoms experienced by patients as seen in the distinct cochlear or vestibular variants of Meniere's disease [38]. Such imaging studies also found a correlation between the progress of the EH imaged with the clinical deterioration of the inner ear functional measurements [39], strengthening the role of hydrops in the pathophysiology of MD.

Measuring the cross-sectional area of the scala media in vivo overcomes the drawbacks of histological shrinking and other artifacts. It has been used in animal models of hydrops with an endolymphatic marker, to study the temporal relation in the development of hydrops, post duct ablation (occurs within days). Functional deficits, measured electrophysiologically (such as cochlear potentials), were surprisingly initially only small changes and most marked at the 8- to 16-week time period when no further hydrops or endolymphatic expansion occurred. The logical extension, if it holds true in humans, would imply that factors apart from or in addition to the hydrops could be responsible for symptoms and relieving the hydrops may not restore normal functioning [40].

Studies determined that the hydrops causes a displacement of the basilar membrane toward the scala tympani which due to anatomical considerations is predominantly at the apex of the cochlea affecting its mechanical-electrical properties. This displacement results in sensorineural hearing loss of frequency below 100 Hz (due to anatomical locations of receptors) which is unlikely to result in clinically appreciated hearing loss, usually tested at frequencies of 250 HZ and higher. Thus, this in endolymphatic hydrops, the pathological findings do not correlate to the low-frequency hearing lost observed in Meniere's disease [41].

12. Hydrops and diagnosis

Given the prevalence of EH in patients of MD, diagnostic tests developed to visualize the EH in vivo have been studied such as gadolinium-based contrast media using heavily T(2)-weighted 3D FLAIR [42]. The advent of such dynamic imaging technologies provides new insights into the pathophysiology of MD such as differential involvement of cochlear and vestibular compartments and the fact that EH occurs in the asymptomatic or unaffected ear with a high (75%)

frequency [38]. Studies also confirm the diagnostic value of such techniques to image the hydrops as essential in the workup of other conditions such as vestibular migraine versus MD [43].

13. Physiology of hydrops and treatment

Most treatment strategies are geared toward the hydrops theory of etiology [44, 45]. Irrespective of the treatment instituted, the success rate of controlling vertigo episodes hovers at 60–80%, strongly suggesting nonspecific therapeutic effect or placebo effect in play. While studies are not always optimally designed with adequate controls; subjective symptoms and the fluctuating nature of the disease itself may compound the results making it difficult to distinguish spontaneous remission versus drug effect versus placebo effects.

Most commonly employed treatments include diuretics and dietary salt restriction which are used based on the rationale of altering the fluid and electrolyte balance; thus decreasing the hydrops, which has shown conflicting results in studies from being effective [46] versus flawed [47].

Several surgical procedures have been devised, such as endolymphatic sac decompressions, shunts and vestibular ablation. The aim of a majority of sac procedures is to decompress the EH and provide a path for drainage. This is conceptually flawed as most shunts created undergo fibrosis and loss of patency and endolymph would not drain into a higher pressure area such as CSF. Ventilation tubes placed in the tympanic membrane were shown to reduce vertigo [48], suggesting that middle ear pressures are involved in the pathophysiology of vertigo. The variable results noted that post-surgery gives credence to the nonspecific placebo effect theory [49].

An interesting result of endolymphatic sac surgery for patients with MD has been the knowledge contributed toward the pathophysiology during revision surgery due to recurrence of symptoms. Extensive granulation tissue and fibrosis found in the mastoid area, in the region of the sac, create a secondary compression coupled with color changes in the implants suggesting that transudative processes in play provide evidence toward endolymphatic malabsorption as the basis of the secondary (induced) MD.

14. Future

Despite advances in technologies, the fundamentals of the pathophysiology in MD remain incomplete. The gaps in knowledge are wide ranging, from natural progression of the disease to etiology, pathophysiology and treatment. To reconcile these controversies, research endeavors should adhere to standardized definitions of MD, selection criteria, control development and results reporting, which will allow comparable analysis across studies.

Animal models and experimental designs more closely reflecting the clinical entity of MD should be the pillar for future research. Overcoming the shortcoming of traditional animal models may allow breakthroughs in answering these questions. Newer models more closely resembling the pathophysiological process in play in MD include mice with vasopressin administration and exploring the role of Latanoprost in MD therapy [50]. Technological advancements in inner ear imaging, histology, immunohistochemistry, genetic testing and functional measurements will allow a more molecular and refined examination of the pathophysiological process.

15. Summary

The pathophysiology of MD remains elusive despite intense research. It is likely that hydrops may not be the cause of MD symptoms, rather an epiphenomenon. Theories on the pathophysiology of MD thus leave several important gaps, mainly around the central theory of EH causing hydrops. They include the following:

- EH cannot comprehensively account for all the physiological changes seen in MD patients.
- EH need not be associated with the characteristic triad of symptoms of MD.
- Several differences exist in the physiological responses in hydropic animals versus MD patients. While this can be accounted for by innate differences between human and animal ears, it is likely related to alternate or additional processes involved in MD.
- The central role played by the endolymphatic sac in the pathophysiology of MD is also challenged, due to the low proportion of hydrops that develops in most animal species following obstruction of the sac and duct. Alternative mechanisms of endolymph production or resorption are likely to be in play in different regions of the labyrinth.

However, given a 100% association of EH in at least one ear of patients with MD, it is likely that EH is more than just an epiphenomenon, rather it is a condition that is necessary but not sufficient for the clinical picture of MD.

Author details

Shazia Mirza* and Sankalp Gokhale

*Address all correspondence to: shazia.mirza@utsouthwestern.edu

UT Southwestern Medical Center, Dallas, Texas, USA

References

[1] Meniere P. Sur une forme de surdité grave dépendant d'une lésion de l'oreille interne. *Gaz Méd de Paris* 1861;16:P29

[2] Merchant, S.N., Adams J.C. and Nadol, J.B., Jr., *Pathophysiology of Meniere's syndrome: are symptoms caused by endolymphatic hydrops?* Otol Neurotol, 2005. **26**(1): p. 74-81.

[3] Morita, N., et al., *Membranous labyrinth volumes in normal ears and Meniere disease: a three-dimensional reconstruction study.* Laryngoscope, 2009. **119**(11): p. 2216-20.

[4] LB, C.B.S.D.N.J.M., *Peripheral vestibular disorders*. Otolaryngol Head Neck Surg, p.2328-45.

[5] Wackym, P.A., et al., *Re-evaluation of the role of the human endolymphatic sac in Meniere's disease*. Otolaryngol Head Neck Surg, 1990. **102**(6): p. 732-44.

[6] Paparella M.M. and Djalilian H.R., *Etiology, pathophysiology of symptoms and pathogenesis of Meniere's disease*. Otolaryngol Clin North Am, 2002. **35**(3): p. 529-45.

[7] Yazawa, Y., et al., *Detection of viral DNA in the endolymphatic sac in Meniere's disease by in situ hybridization*. ORL J Otorhinolaryngol Relat Spec, 2003. **65**(3): p. 162-8.

[8] Vrabec, J.T., *Herpes simplex virus and Meniere's disease*. Laryngoscope, 2003. **113**(9): p. 1431-8.

[9] Pulec, J.L., *Meniere's disease of syphilitic etiology*. Ear Nose Throat J, 1997. **76**(8): p. 508-10, 512 514, passim.

[10] Requena, T., et al., *Familial clustering and genetic heterogeneity in Meniere's disease*. Clin Genet, 2014. **85**(3): p. 245-52.

[11] Requena, T., et al., *Identification of two novel mutations in FAM136A and DTNA genes in autosomal-dominant familial Meniere's disease*. Hum Mol Genet, 2015. **24**(4): p. 1119-26.

[12] Adams, J.C., *Clinical implications of inflammatory cytokines in the cochlea: a technical note*. Otol Neurotol, 2002. **23**(3): p. 316-22.

[13] Yamane, H., et al., *Assessment of Meniere's disease from a radiological aspect - saccular otoconia as a cause of Meniere's disease?* Acta Otolaryngol, 2012. **132**(10): p. 1054-60.

[14] Paparella, M.M., de Sousa L.C. and Mancini F., *Meniere's syndrome and otitis media*. Laryngoscope, 1983. **93**(11 Pt 1): p. 1408-15.

[15] Segal, S., et al., *Is there a relation between acoustic trauma or noise-induced hearing loss and a subsequent appearance of Meniere's disease? An epidemiologic study of 17245 cases and a review of the literature*. Otol Neurotol, 2003. **24**(3): p. 387-91.

[16] Yoon, T.H., Paparella, M.M. and Schachern P.A., *Otosclerosis involving the vestibular aqueduct and Meniere's disease*. Otolaryngol Head Neck Surg, 1990. **103**(1): p. 107-12.

[17] Nakashima, T., et al., *A perspective from magnetic resonance imaging findings of the inner ear: Relationships among cerebrospinal, ocular and inner ear fluids*. Auris Nasus Larynx, 2012. **39**(4): p. 345-55.

[18] Teranishi, M., et al., *Polymorphisms in genes involved in the free-radical process in patients with sudden sensorineural hearing loss and Meniere's disease*. Free Radic Res, 2013. **47**(6-7): p. 498-506.

[19] Takeda, T., et al., *Hormonal aspects of Meniere's disease on the basis of clinical and experimental studies*. ORL J Otorhinolaryngol Relat Spec, 2010. **71 Suppl 1**: p. 1-9.

[20] Silverstein, H. and Takeda T., *Endolymphatic sac obstruction. Biochemical studies*. Ann Otol Rhinol Laryngol, 1977. **86**(4 Pt 1): p. 493-9.

[21] Keithley, E.M., Horowitz, S. and Ruckenstein, M.J., *Na,K-ATPase in the cochlear lateral wall of human temporal bones with endolymphatic hydrops.* Ann Otol Rhinol Laryngol, 1995. **104**(11): p. 858-63.

[22] Yoon, T.H., et al., *Cellular changes in Reissner's membrane in endolymphatic hydrops.* Ann Otol Rhinol Laryngol, 1991. **100**(4 Pt 1): p. 288-93.

[23] Andrews, J.C., Bohmer, A. and Hoffman, L.F., *The measurement and manipulation of intra-labyrinthine pressure in experimental endolymphatic hydrops.* Laryngoscope, 1991. **101**(6 Pt 1): p. 661-8.

[24] Nakashima, T. and Ito, A., *Effect of increased perilymphatic pressure on endocochlear potential.* Ann Otol Rhinol Laryngol, 1981. **90**(3 Pt 1): p. 264-6.

[25] Rosingh, H.J., Wit, H.P. and Albers, F.W., *Perilymphatic pressure dynamics following posture change in patients with Meniere's disease and in normal hearing subjects.* Acta Otolaryngol, 1998. **118**(1): p. 1-5.

[26] Warmerdam, T.J., et al., *Perilymphatic and endolymphatic pressures during endolymphatic hydrops.* Eur Arch Otorhinolaryngol, 2003. **260**(1): p. 9-11.

[27] Rosingh, H.J., Wit, H.P. and Albers, F.W., *Non-invasive perilymphatic pressure measurement in patients with Meniere's disease.* Clin Otolaryngol Allied Sci, 1996. **21**(4): p. 335-8.

[28] Brown, D.J., et al., *Changes in cochlear function during acute endolymphatic hydrops development in guinea pigs.* Hear Res, 2013. **296**: p. 96-106.

[29] Nadol, J.B., Jr., *Positive Hennebert's sign in Meniere's disease.* Arch Otolaryngol, 1977. **103**(9): p. 524-30.

[30] Rizvi, S.S., *Investigations into the cause of canal paresis in Meniere's disease.* Laryngoscope, 1986. **96**(11): p. 1258-71.

[31] Nadol, J.B., Jr. and Thornton, A.R., *Ultrastructural findings in a case of Meniere's disease.* Ann Otol Rhinol Laryngol, 1987. **96**(4): p. 449-54.

[32] Futaki, T., Kitahara, M. and Morimoto, M., *A comparison of the furosemide and glycerol tests for Meniere's disease. With special reference to the bilateral lesion.* Acta Otolaryngol, 1977. **83**(3-4): p. 272-8.

[33] Brookes, G.B., Morrison, A.W. and Richard, R., *Otoadmittance changes following glycerol dehydration in Meniere's disease.* Acta Otolaryngol, 1984. **98**(1-2): p. 30-41.

[34] Di Girolamo, S., et al., *Postural control and glycerol test in Meniere's disease.* Acta Otolaryngol, 2001. **121**(7): p. 813-7.

[35] Ferraro, J.A. and Krishnan, G., *Cochlear potentials in clinical audiology.* Audiol Neurotol, 1997. **2**(5): p. 241-56.

[36] Sperling, N.M., et al., *Symptomatic versus asymptomatic endolymphatic hydrops: a histopathologic comparison.* Laryngoscope, 1993. **103**(3): p. 277-85.

[37] Silverstein, H., *The effects of perfusing the perilymphatic space with artificial endolymph.* Ann Otol Rhinol Laryngol, 1970. **79**(4): p. 754-65.

[38] Pyykko, I., et al., *Meniere's disease: a reappraisal supported by a variable latency of symptoms and the MRI visualisation of endolymphatic hydrops.* BMJ Open, 2013;3:e001555 doi:10.1136/bmjopen-2012-001555

[39] Gurkov, R., et al., *In vivo visualized endolymphatic hydrops and inner ear functions in patients with electrocochleographically confirmed Meniere's disease.* Otol Neurotol, 2012. **33**(6): p. 1040-5.

[40] Salt, A.N. and DeMott, J., *Time course of endolymph volume increase in experimental hydrops measured in vivo with an ionic volume marker.* Hear Res, 1994. **74**(1-2): p. 165-72.

[41] Nageris, B., Adams, J.C. and Merchant, S.N., *A human temporal bone study of changes in the basilar membrane of the apical turn in endolymphatic hydrops.* Am J Otol, 1996. **17**(2): p. 245-52.

[42] Naganawa, S., et al., *Visualization of endolymphatic hydrops in Meniere's disease with single-dose intravenous gadolinium-based contrast media using heavily T(2)-weighted 3D-FLAIR.* Magn Reson Med Sci, 2010. **9**(4): p. 237-42.

[43] Gurkov, R., et al., *Endolymphatic hydrops in patients with vestibular migraine and auditory symptoms.* Eur Arch Otorhinolaryngol, 2014. **271**(10): p. 2661-7.

[44] Thomsen, J., *Defining valid approaches to therapy for Meniere's disease.* Ear Nose Throat J, 1986. **65**(9): p. 10-8.

[45] Torok, N., *Old and new in Meniere disease.* Laryngoscope, 1977. **87**(11): p. 1870-7.

[46] van Deelen, G.W. and Huizing, E.H., *Use of a diuretic (Dyazide) in the treatment of Meniere's disease. A double-blind cross-over placebo-controlled study.* ORL J Otorhinolaryngol Relat Spec, 1986. **48**(5): p. 287-92.

[47] Ruckenstein, M.J., Rutka, J.A. and Hawke, M., *The treatment of Meniere's disease: Torok revisited.* Laryngoscope, 1991. **101**(2): p. 211-8.

[48] Montandon, P., Guillemin, P. and Hausler, R., *Prevention of vertigo in Meniere's syndrome by means of transtympanic ventilation tubes.* ORL J Otorhinolaryngol Relat Spec, 1988. **50**(6): p. 377-81.

[49] Bretlau, P., et al., *Placebo effect in surgery for Meniere's disease: nine-year follow-up.* Am J Otol, 1989. **10**(4): p. 259-61.

[50] Katagiri, Y., et al., *Long-term administration of vasopressin can cause Meniere's disease in mice.* Acta Otolaryngol, 2014. **134**(10): p. 990-1004.

Section 5

Ménière's Disease - Audiological and Vestibular Evaluation

Chapter 6

Audiological Assessment in Meniere's Disease

Dinesh Kumar Sharma

Additional information is available at the end of the chapter

http://dx.doi.org/10.5772/66486

Abstract

Meniere's disease is a progressive disorder characterized by recurrent episodes of spontaneous vertigo, sensorineural hearing loss and tinnitus, often with a feeling of fullness in the ear. The exact ethology is not known. In 1972, a diagnostic criterion for Meniere's disease was proposed by American Academy of Otolaryngology-Head and Neck Surgery (AAO-HNS), and till date, it has been revised twice in the years 1985 and 1995. The principal audiological investigation is pure tone audiometry combined with a glycerol test. Speech audiometry and otoacoustic emissions also play a limited role. The value of electrocochleography is limited.

Keywords: pure tone audiometry, glycerol test, speech audiometry, OAE, electrocochleography

1. Introduction

Meniere's disease named after an Italian scientist, Prosper Meniere, is a progressive disorder characterized by recurrent episodes of spontaneous vertigo, sensorineural hearing loss and tinnitus, often with a feeling of fullness in the ear [1]. The characteristic of the disease is that it is an unpredictable, fluctuating illness with noteworthy hidden disability [2].

The precise cause of Meniere's disease is still being investigated. It is believed to be associated with endolymphatic hydrops, that is, raised endolymph pressure in the membranous labyrinth of the inner ear, which gets dilated like a balloon when pressure increases and drainage is blocked. This results in swelling of the endolymphatic sac and other tissues in the vestibular system (responsible for the body's sense of balance), creating an acute vestibular imbalance, resulting in vertigo and fluctuating hearing loss [3].

Another suggested etiology is the autoimmune nature of the disease. The idea of autoimmunity was brought forward when improvement in bilateral progressive sensorineural hearing

INTECH
open science | open minds

© 2017 The Author(s). Licensee InTech. This chapter is distributed under the terms of the Creative Commons Attribution License (http://creativecommons.org/licenses/by/3.0), which permits unrestricted use, distribution, and reproduction in any medium, provided the original work is properly cited.

loss was recorded following immunosuppressive therapy. The studies of the human endolymphatic sac have also suggested that it is the primary immunocompetent structure in the inner ear, which is capable of processing antigen, synthesizing antibodies and raising a cellular immune response [4].

No single test that makes the diagnosis of Meniere's disease with conformity has been established. Complete history, including a detailed description of the pattern of disease presentation supported by quantitative testing, helps in arriving at a diagnosis [5].

A number of international interdisciplinary organizations in a consensus paper have drawn diagnostic criteria for Meniere's disease. The paper suggests two categories of the Meniere's disease, definite and probable. The definition of definite variety incorporates a clinical criteria and observation of episodes of vertigo associated with audiometric findings of sensorineural hearing loss involving low and middle frequencies and triad of symptoms that include fluctuant hearing loss, tinnitus and/or fullness of the involved ear. The criteria limit the duration of vertigo from 20 min to 12 h. The definition of probable variety of Meniere's disease encompasses vertigo or dizziness and extends to episodic ear-related symptoms, which may occur for a variable period time between 20 min and 24 h [2].

The natural history of Meniere's disease is inconstant but usually progressive. The classical triad of tinnitus or aural fullness with episodic vertigo and hearing impairment is often not seen at the beginning of the disease. The disease starts as a single symptom entity, and only cochlear symptoms occur at the first stage. The period between the primary symptoms and the manifestation of other symptoms varies from months to several years with an estimated average of 6–18 months. After this period of variable duration, the complete triad of symptoms will appear [6].

Episodic attacks of vertigo (so-called Meniere's attack) are the most troublesome of the symptoms to the patient, and it is usually the symptom that causes the patient to seek medical treatment. The vertigo patient perceives either that the world is spinning around them or that they themselves are spinning. Typically, it occurs in the form of a series of attacks over a period of weeks or months, interspersed by periods of remission of variable duration [7].

When the patient experiences a feeling of rotation, the sign is nystagmus, which has been described as a condition of involuntary movements of eyeball. This is accompanied by other symptoms such as giddiness and sweating [8].

On most occasions, patients experience a heaviness or fullness of the involved ear, which is accompanied by impairment of hearing and ringing sensation. Often the beginning of symptoms is precipitous, which reaches its zenith within a span of minutes to hours. The entire episode persists for an hour so before it wanes. The patient may experience unsteadiness for a couple of hours or days after the attack subsides. In between episodes of the disease, subjects may suffer from positional vertigo [9].

Vertigo is the most disabling one among the cardinal symptoms of the disease. It adversely affects almost every aspect of life disturbing the normal lifestyle of the patient. The vertigo is made worse especially when movement is involved. Patient's ability to lead a normal way life is hampered by risks of fall. The chances of such events are made worse by small head movements, which make the patient subjectively very "ill." Vertigo can completely undermine the individual. This leads the patients to confine themselves to bed until the symptoms improve [10].

Some sufferers experience "drop attacks," which are sudden, severe unexplained falls without loss of consciousness or associated vertigo. These drop attacks are due to acute utriculosaccular dysfunction and are triggered by changes in inner ear pressure affecting otolith function [11].

Another unusual pattern of clinical presentation has been described, known as Lermoyez attacks. As opposed to typical spells in which tinnitus and hearing loss precede and worsen with the onset of vertigo, in Lermoyez attacks increased tinnitus and hearing loss precede the vertiginous episode and dramatically resolve with onset of vertigo [12].

Tinnitus experienced by Meniere's patients is continual and does not abate with time, although its intensity may vary. In addition, it may be heard more as a loud roaring or buzzing sensation, rather than a whistling, and is most commonly non-pulsatile and of the low-frequency type. The pitch tends to be related to the region of the most severe hearing loss and the magnitude of tinnitus roughly proportional to the severity of hearing loss [13].

A sensation of aural fullness that may precede a definite vertiginous spell, is considered a symptom alternative to tinnitus in the criteria of AAO-HNS (1985, 1995) and is experienced by 74.1% of the patients [14].

The hearing loss usually affects one ear, which typically loses sensitivity to low-frequency sounds and is of sensorineural type. As the hearing thresholds rise, dynamic range decreases, the sounds are typically described as "tinny" by the patient, the quality of sounds becomes poor, and loudness of loud sounds rises rapidly due to a phenomenon known as recruitment. The patients become intolerant to such loud sounds. During the early days of the disease, the hearing loss tends to return to within normal thresholds, and however, later in course of disease, hearing loss persists and even deteriorates over the course of following episodes. Even in terms of frequency involvement, the hearing loss spreads to involve all the frequencies showing a flat line on the audiogram. The sensorineural hearing loss in Meniere's disease involves low frequencies giving a flat audiometric pattern, but sometimes we get peak audiograms that are nearly normal hearing at around 2 kHz and decreased sensorineural hearing at lower and higher frequencies. This type of pattern is considered to be diagnostic of Meniere's disease and is more commonly seen in patients with disease of short duration. Over time, the hearing loss flattens and becomes less variable [15].

Patients become profoundly deaf rarely in 1–2% of severely affected patients [2].

Additional features are diplacusis that is unusual sensitivity to noises, sounds can seem tinny or distorted known as dysacusis, a difference in the perception of pitch between the ears (43.6%) and recruitment (56%) [16].

2. Investigations used to support the diagnosis of Meniere's disease

As of now, no single test can claim to make a reliable diagnosis of Meniere's disease; rather it is based on a complete history with a detailed description of the pattern of disease presentation, supported by quantitative testing.

In 1972, a diagnostic criterion for Meniere's disease was proposed by American Academy of Otolaryngology-Head and Neck Surgery (AAO-HNS), and till date, it has been revised twice in the years 1985 and 1995 [5].

The latest criteria used for diagnosis of Meniere's disease are the one proposed by AAO-HNS in the year 1995 [5].

AAO-HNS (1995) also introduced a staging system for cases of definite Meniere's disease. Staging is based solely on hearing, which is the most readily measurable variable and most closely related to the natural history of the disease [17].

Stages 1 and 2 are considered representative of early reversible disease that is susceptible to remission, whereas stages 3 and 4 are considered fixed or not reversible.

A good classic history with the criteria as outlined by AAO-HNS is adequate for diagnosing a case of Meniere's disease.

2.1. Pure tone audiometry (PTA).

PTA is the elementary investigation for reaching at a diagnosis and following up the patient during the course of treatment. A four-tone average of 0.5, 1, 2 and 3 kHz has been adopted in the guidelines of AAO-HNS (1985, 1995), and a change of 10 dB or more in PTA or a greater than 15% change in word recognition score is considered a clinically significant change during diagnosis and treatment [5].

Pure tone audiometry is the primary tool applied by the clinicians to ascertain hearing thresholds of the patient. It is used to document the degree and type of auditory impairment. These elements along with shape of the audiogram lay the ground for designing and implementing a line of treatment. This investigation is principally used in adults and grown-up children as PTA is dependent on patient's cooperation and his/her response to the pure tone signals [7].

Pure tone audiometry has assumed an established role in diagnosis of hearing impairment. Pre-calibrated pure tones are presented to the patient in sound-treated chambers. Circumaural headphones, insert phones and bone oscillators are used to deliver these tones to patient to determine air-conduction and bone-conduction thresholds across a frequency range from 250 to 8000 Hz. The thresholds are recorded in terms of decibel HL. Specific algorithms are available to determine need for masking the non-test ear when asymmetrical hearing presents the risk of cross hearing. Procedures and formulae are available to calculate the initial masking levels needed both for air-conduction and for masking levels to determine masked thresholds. The thresholds so detected are plotted on an audiogram using standardized symbols. Air-conduction thresholds tell about the degree, and bone-conduction thresholds convey type of hearing loss.

Apart from the degree of hearing loss, the pattern of audiogram tells about the type of hearing loss, whether it is conductive, sensorineural or mixed. Pure tone audiometry is regarded by some as initial screening test of choice for audiological dysfunction [18].

Staging of Definite Meniere's disease may be done in all the patients on the basic degree of hearing loss.

Stage	Four-tone average (dB) (0.5, 1, 2 and 3 kHz)
1	<25
2	26–40
3	41–70
4	>70

The hearing loss in Meniere's disease is unilateral in about 70–85% of cases. However, the incidence of bilaterality increases with the duration of the disease, reaching about 40% after 15 years [19].

Audiograms are performed at different points during the course or progression of disease, and the hearing loss shows a fluctuating pattern. During the initial stages of the disease, if the PTA is performed after an episode has subsided, the audiogram may look to be normal. As the patient continues to experience more and more attacks, some degree of hearing loss tends to persist in between the attacks. However, in the later stages of the disease, the hearing loss establishes as non-fluctuating and permanent [20].

In the early stages of Meniere's disease, the characteristic audiometric configuration is a rising curve, that is, as the frequency increases, the hearing loss decreases. This contour has also been called a "reverse slope" audiogram, since high-frequency losses are by far the most frequent pattern in the hearing-impaired population. Word recognition (discrimination) has been reported in some studies as poor as 32%. Although mid- and high-frequency sensitivity tends to be good in the early stages, as the disease progresses, these frequencies become involved, leaving the patient with a "flat" audiometric configuration. The hearing loss may progress to a profoundly impaired degree as the disease process continues. However, the degree of hearing loss seldom exceeds a 70 dB average [21].

There is no classical audiogram pattern that can be used to identify Meniere's disease. However, there are certain features that have been commonly observed. These include:

- A varying degree of sensorineural hearing loss.
- This hearing loss is usually low frequency.
- The audiogram may be "flat," upward sloping or downward sloping.

In a study of 211 consecutive patients with classic Meniere's disease, the audiological pattern was flat in 42%, peaked type in 32%, downward sloping in 19% and rising in 7% patients [22].

In a study conducted in our department, 31 patients of either sex between the age group of 18 and 65 years presenting with history of attacks of vertigo, accompanied with tinnitus, sensorineural hearing loss and aural fullness were selected randomly; 64% of these patients had either a flat audiometric graph or a low-frequency hearing loss as evidenced by downward sloping audiometric pattern. In this study, in 18 patients, the duration of symptoms was less than 12 months. In these 18 patients, 29 ears were affected; of these, 45% ears had rising or peak type of audiograms. Further analysis of the audiometric pattern in this study revealed that in patients with sudden onset of symptoms, 50% ears showed either a rising or a peak type of graph. On the contrary, among those patients with gradual onset of symptoms, 76% ears showed a flat or sloping type of graph. This correlates with the findings of a study which concluded that rising or peak audiograms appear more commonly in patients with disease of short duration [23].

In a study comprising of 111 patients with Meniere's disease, pure tone and speech audiometry was performed. The affected ears showed reduced hearing in both the modalities. An objective classification method used to determine audiogram shape indicated that affected ears more frequently show "low" or "low + high" hearing losses. The study concluded that shape of hearing loss does not depend on duration of affection of disease [24].

2.2. Short increment sensitivity index test (SISI)

It is a useful test in distinguishing between cochlear and retro-cochlear lesion. It determines the capacity of a patient to detect a brief 1 dB increment at a 20 dB supra-threshold tone (called carrier tone) in various frequencies (preferably at 1000 and 4000 Hz). If SISI score is above 70%, it is considered as positive SISI and pathology lies in the cochlea. If SISI score is <30%, it is negative SISI and here pathology lies elsewhere than inner ear [18].

On the basis of PTA report, all the patients suffering from sensorineural hearing loss may further be subjected to glycerol test.

2.3. Glycerol test

The assumption that an increase in endolymph volume, with its effect on labyrinthine membrane behavior producing in part, the hearing loss and vestibular deficit in Meniere's disease has led to the administration of dehydrating agents like glycerol. The goal is to reduce the volume abnormalities in inner ear and produce a measurable change in response that is improvement in behavioral audiometric test scores.

Glycerol, a potent osmolar agent, elevates osmotic pressure of the liquid in which it is dissolved. In the cochlear context, upon administration to a patient it lowers the volume of membranous labyrinth. Animal studies in which endolymphatic hydrops was induced surgically, responded to glycerol through intracellular and extracellular edema. The increased secretion of glycoproteins following administration of glycerol induces endolymph flow into endolymphatic sac. Thus, glycerol promotes the absorption of endolymph both in radial and in longitudinal directions [25]. This is a simple and rapid method that provides information on the cochlear response to the osmotic changes produced by glycerol in the inner ear.

Glycerol is administered orally to patients to reduce fluid abnormalities in the inner ear. It affects hearing temporarily (for a few hours), the results of which are measured by audiogram.

2.4. Method of glycerol test

The patients are advised to report empty stomach on the day of investigation. PTA test is performed before the administration of glycerol and then patient is administered a solution of 86% of glycerol (1.5 mg/kg of body weight) dissolved in equal volume of physiological saline.

Pure tone audiometry is then repeated at 1, 2 and 3 hours of glycerol administration.

The glycerol test is regarded as positive:

- When the hearing threshold is lowered at least 15 dB at minimum three frequencies or
- When there is a total pure tone threshold shift of 25 dB at three consecutive frequencies or
- When there is a 16% improvement in speech discrimination [26, 27].

In the study conducted at our department (whose results have yet to be published), only those patients were included who had definite Meniere's disease based on the AAO-HNS criteria. All these patients were subjected to glycerol testing to determine their suitability for administration of hydrochlorothiazide. In this study, 74% of patients had a positive glycerol test.

Another study has reported its experience of using the glycerol test in 122 patients with combination of sensorineural hearing loss, tinnitus or vestibular symptoms, in which endolymphatic hydrops was considered a possibility. Fifty percent of patients ultimately were found to have endolymphatic hydrops and positive test [28].

In a study of series of 95 patients with Meniere's disease, 47% were found to have a positive glycerol dehydration test. Yet another study reported that 60% of patients with Meniere's disease have positive tests. This study also noted that positive tests were found only in ears with Meniere's disease [29]. In another study, intravenous administration of glycerol was performed instead of oral administration. Positive results were obtained in 50% (15 out of 30) of patients 1 hour after administration. The positive ratio was same as oral glycerol test [30]. Thus, the results of glycerol testing in our study are comparable with other studies. The relatively higher percentage of positive glycerol test in our study could be due to the fact that subjects included in our study met the criteria of "definite Meniere's disease" as laid down by AAO-HNS. In our study, the results of administration of hydrochlorothiazide to patients who tested positive on glycerol testing indicate an across the board improvement in symptoms of Meniere's disease at the end of follow-up. Thus, it may be concluded that glycerol testing in patients with "definite Meniere's disease" as assessed by AAO-HNS criteria is a good idea to select patients who will respond to administration of osmotic diuretics.

Most patients may suffer headache and nausea after drinking the glycerol for post-glycerol audiometric evaluation, which usually subsides after few hours.

3. Speech audiometry

The objective of speech audiometry testing is to measure patient's ability to identify speech stimuli, to confirm results of pure tone audiometry and to rule out the presence of nonorganic hearing loss or retro-cochlear pathology.

The battery of speech audiometry tests includes speech detection threshold (SDT), speech recognition threshold (SRT) and word recognition score (WRS).

Word recognition test scores are often plotted on a graph. A point on this graph represents the percentage words correctly repeated by the patient at a specified intensity level from completed standardized list of words. Cochlear pathology tends to demonstrate a "plateau effect," reaching a ceiling of performance at <100% and no improvement in the score despite a rise in intensity.

4. Otoacoustic emission

An otoacoustic emission (OAE) is a low-level sound emitted by the cochlea either spontaneously or evoked by an auditory stimulus. Specifically, OAEs provide information related to the function of the outer hair cells (OHC) [31].

The use of OAEs in the assessment of patients with Meniere's disease has been well documented. According to Van Hufflen et al., patients with Meniere's disease can essentially be divided into four categories. It has been documented that OAEs present in ears with minimal hearing loss and absent in ears where pure tone thresholds exceed 60 dB HL. Both these scenarios are acceptable clinically. Among patients who have hearing thresholds in intermediate range of 30–60 dB HL two scenarios emerge. In the first scenario, OAEs are measurable in large values, while OAEs are not measurable at all. It has been postulated that variable patterns of OAEs in patients with Meniere's disease may be due to more than one precise sites of lesion. It was postulated by Hall that among patients in whom OAEs are present despite a hearing impairment more than 30 dB, the audiometric picture is not representing outer hair cells. He said that in these patients, the outer hair cells may have been spared and data are representative of inner hair cell function [32].

A number of studies have been conducted to determine the utility of OAE and changes in OAE during glycerol test undertaken to diagnose endolymphatic hydrops. In a study, TEOAE and DPOAE were measured before and 3 h after oral administration of glycerol in 22 years of patients with Meniere's disease. The positive result in the glycerol test was observed in 11 of 22 ears. However, of the two OAEs, DPOAE was considered more appropriate than TEOAE for monitoring during the glycerol test because of its high sensitivity in detection of changes in cochlear function. The study concluded that clinical use of OAE, especially DPOAE, as a test complementary to pure tone audiometry during the glycerol test is very useful and will improve the diagnosis of endolymphatic hydrops [33].

The worth of DPOAE to spot minimal inner ear dysfunction which might be due to endolymphatic hydrops and may otherwise go undetected on pure tone testing has been emphasized by a few clinical studies. A study specifically examined a set of patients whose only presenting complaint was fullness of ear/ears. The study used glycerol test with PTA and DPOAE to diagnose subjects at an early stage of Meniere's disease and may have the potential to progress toward the full-blown disease. It was concluded that those patients in whom the only symptom is fullness of ear/ears may potentially be in early stages of the condition [34].

A study was conducted to follow up the dynamics of pure tone threshold and DPOAE amplitude changes induced by glycerol with reference to its activity in inner ear; 38 patients with Meniere's disease and having positive glycerol test were included in the study. It was concluded that audiometry and DPOAE measurements in the glycerol test procedure are the most profitable after the third hour since glycerol administration due to the most significant outcomes of both at this time. Observed changes in pure tone audiometry concern lower frequencies and in DPOAE middle frequencies [25].

5. Electrocochleography

"Electrocochleography" (ECochG) is an investigation employed to measure electrical potentials of cochlea. The components of ECochG include measurement of cochlear potentials in response to a stimulus and measurement of the whole nerve or compound action potential (AP) of the eighth nerve.

A study conducted to evaluate the role of ECochG in the diagnosis of Meniere's disease concluded that ECochG has little role in diagnosing or ruling out Meniere's disease [35].

Although the utility of ECochG diagnosis continues to be disputed, it has been proposed that in the situation that ECochG confirms the diagnosis of Meniere's disease, one can be confident in deciding about an invasive therapy. What course be adopted when patient exhibits symptoms that confirm the diagnosis of Meniere's disease, but ECochG is within normal limits remains a dilemma [36].

6. Conclusion

It is a challenging task to arrive at a conclusive diagnosis of Meniere's disease. A detailed history must be elicited from the patients, who should be encouraged to describe the symptoms in their own language. The sequence of events as they appeared and their characteristics help in arriving at a possible diagnosis. A thorough clinical examination is a mandatory component of initial encounter with the patient. Pure tone audiometry is the principal tool to document nature and degree of hearing loss. It is highly useful to have previous audiograms and compare them with the current audiogram. It helps understand fluctuant nature of disease and its progression. Glycerol test is a useful component of audiological assessment and has been combined with PTA and OAE. In author's experience, results of glycerol test in combination with PTA may be used to decide the possible line of treatment. Those patients with a positive glycerol test give better results with diuretics such as hydrochlorothiazide and those with a negative test respond better to oral steroids such as prednisolone. The word recognition scores recorded in speech audiometry demonstrate a typical "plateau effect," reaching a ceiling of performance at <100% and no improvement in the score despite a rise in intensity. OAE, especially DPOAE, has been particularly found useful in diagnosis of Meniere's disease. The role of electrocochleography (ECochG) in the diagnosis and monitoring of treatment for Meniere's disease remains controversial.

Author details

Dinesh Kumar Sharma

Address all correspondence to: dr.dineshkumar@gmail.com

Department of ENT, Government Medical College, Amritsar, India

References

[1] Arenberg IK, Wells JA, Shambaugh GE. Definitions and semantics: an overview of Meniere's disease and endolymphatic hydrops. In: Arenberg IK (ed.) Surgery of the inner ear, Kugler Publications, Amsterdam, 1991, pp. 3-7.

[2] Anderson JP, Harris JP. Impact of Meniere's disease on quality of life. Otol Neurotol 2001;22(6):888-894.

[3] Kawauchi H. Distribution of immunocompetent cells in the endolymphatic sac. Ann Otol Rhinol Laryngol 1992;10:39-47.

[4] Bronstein A. Visual symptoms and vertigo. Neurol Clin 2005;23(3):705-713.

[5] AAO-HNS 1995 committee on hearing and equilibrium guidelines for the diagnosis and evaluation of therapy in Meniere's disease. Otolaryngol Head Neck Surg 1995;113:181-185.

[6] Tokomasu K, Fujino A, Naganuma H, Hoshino I, Arai M. Initial symptoms and retrospective analysis of prognosis in Meniere's disease. Acta Otolaryngol (Stockh) 1996;524:43-49.

[7] Gibson WPR, Arenberg IK. The mechanism which cause the vertigo in Meniere's disease. In: Sterkers O, Ferrary E, Dauman R, Sauvage JP, Tran Ba Huy P (Eds) Meniere's disease 1999—Update, Kugler Publications, The Hague, The Netherlands, 2000, pp. 451-454.

[8] Bance M. The changing direction of nystagmus in acute Meniere's disease: pathophysiological implications. Laryngoscope 1991;(101):197-201.

[9] Mizukoshi K, Watanabe Y, Shojaku H, Matsunaga T, Tokumasu K. Preliminary guidelines for reporting treatment results in Meniere's disease conducted by the committee of the Japanese Society for equilibrium research. Acta Otolaryngol (Stockh) 1993;519:211-215.

[10] Cohen H, Ewell LR, Jenkins HA. Disability in Meniere's disease. Arch Otolaryngol Head Neck Surg 1995;121:29-33.

[11] Baloh RW, Jacobson K, Winder T. Drop attacks with Meniere's syndrome. Ann Neurol 1990;28 (3):384-387.

[12] Schmidt RII, Schoonhaven R. Lermoyez's syndrome: a follow-up study in 12 patients. Acta Otolaryngol (Stockh) 1989;107:467-473.

[13] Vernon J, Johnson R, Schleuning A. The characteristics and natural history of tinnitus in Meniere's disease. Otolaryngol Clin Am 1980;13(4):611-619.

[14] Paparella MM, Djalilian HR. Etiology, pathophysiology of symptoms, and pathogenesis of Meniere's disease. Otolaryngol Clin North Am 2002;35(3):529-545.

[15] Sakurai T, Yamane H, Nakai Y. Some aspects of hearing change in Meniere's patients. Acta Otolaryngol Suppl 1991;486:492.

[16] Paparella MM. The cause (multifactorial inheritance) and pathogenesis (endolymphatic malabsorption) of Meniere's disease and its symptoms (mechanical and chemical). Acta Otolaryngol (Stockh) 1985;99:445-451.

[17] Thirlwall AS, Kundu S. Diuretics for Ménière's disease or syndrome. Cochrane Database of Syst Rev 2006;3:CD003599.

[18] Lovrinic JH. Pure tone and speech audiometry. In: Keith RW, editor. Audiology for the physician, 1980. pp. 13-31. Baltimore: Williams and Wilkins.

[19] Morrison A. The surgery of vertigo: sassus drainage for idiopathic endolymphatic hydrops. J Laryngol Otol 1976;90:87-93.

[20] Melville da Cruz. Ménière's disease: a stepwise approach. Med Today 2014;15(3):18-26

[21] Accessed online at http://www.audiology.org/sites/default/files/journal/JAAA_17_01_Editorial.pdf.

[22] Meyerhoff WL, Paparella MM, Gudbrandsson FK. Clinical evaluation of Ménière's disease. Laryngoscope. 1981;91(10):1663-1668.

[23] Paparella MM, Griebie MS. Bilaterality of Meniere's disease. Acta Otolaryngol 1984;97:233-237.

[24] Mateijsen DJ, Van Hengel PW, Van Huffelen WM, Wit HP, Albers FW. Pure-tone and speech audiometry in patients with Menière's disease. Clin Otolaryngol Allied Sci. 2001;26(5):379-87.

[25] Jablonka-Strom A, Pospiech L, Zatonski M, Bochnia M. Dynamics of pure tone audiometry and DPOAE changes induced by glycerol in Meniere's disease. Eur Arch Otorhinolaryngol. 2013;270(5):1751-1756. Published online 2012 Nov 16. doi:10.1007/s00405-012-2246-6. PMCID: PMC3624005.

[26] Aso S. The intravenously administered glycerol test. Acta Otolaryngol (Stockh) Suppl 1993;504:51-54.

[27] Klockhoff I. Diagnosis of Meniere's disease. Arch Otorhinolaryngol 1976;212:309-314.

[28] Snyder JM. Extensive use of a diagnostic test for Meniere disease. Arch Otolaryngol. 1974;100(5):360-365.

[29] Stahle J, Klockhoff I. Diagnostic procedures, differential diagnosis, and general conclusions. In: Controversial Aspects of Meniere Disease. CR Pfaltz (ed.), Thieme Inc., New York, NY, 1986, pp. 71-86.

[30] Tooru S, Akiko S, Fumio S, Hiroya F, Masafumi S. Intravenous glycerol test for Meniere's disease. Equilib Res 1999; 58:36-39.

[31] Stach B. Comprehensive dictionary of audiology illustrated. 2nd ed. New York: Thomson Delmar Learning; 2003.

[32] Accessed online at http://www.audiologyonline.com/articles/otoacoustic-emissions-beyond-newborn-hearing-838.

[33] Sakashita T, Kubo T, Kyunai K, Ueno K, Hikawa C, Shibata T, Yamane H, Kusuki M, Wada T, Uyama T. Changes in otoacoustic emission during the glycerol test in the ears of patients with Meniere's disease. Nihon Jibiinkoka Gakkai Kaiho. 2001;104(6):682-93.

[34] Magliulo G, Cianfrone G, Triches L, Altissimi G, D'Amico R. Distortion-product otoacoustic emissions and glycerol testing in endolymphatic hydrops. Laryngoscope. 2001;111(1):102-9.

[35] Kim HH, Kumar A, Battista RA, Wiet RJ. Electrocochleography in patients with Meniere's disease. Am J Otolaryngol. 2005;26(2):128-31.

[36] Linda T. Nguyen, Jeffrey P. Harris, Quyen T. Nguyen. Clinical utility of electrocochleography in the diagnosis and management of Meniere's disease: AOS and ANS Membership Survey Data. Otol Neurotol. 2010;31(3):455-459. doi:10.1097/MAO.0b013e3181d2779c

Chapter 7

Electrophysiology in Ménière's Disease

Pauliana Lamounier

Additional information is available at the end of the chapter

http://dx.doi.org/10.5772/intechopen.69668

Abstract

Ménière's disease (MD) is a progressive inner ear disorder that affects at least 0.2% of the population in EUA. The symptoms triad of fluctuating hearing loss, tinnitus, and vertigo was described by Prosper Ménière for more than a century and its pathophysiology is still unknown. MD has a fluctuating course and in many cases, difficult clinical management. Progressive hearing loss and intense dizzying seizures becomes more frequent as the disease progresses. All of this increases the challenges of accurate identification and has probably led to the trial of several tests for identifying MD. The tests are useful tools to assist the otolaryngologist both in diagnosis and prognosis of MD. These tests includes audiometry, otoacustic emission (OAE), electrocochleography (EcochG), vestibular evoked myogenic potentials (VEMP), cochlear hydrops analysis masking procedure (CHAMP) and video head impulse test (vHIT).

Keywords: Meniere's disease, endolymphatic hydrops, electrocochleography, VEMP, CHAMP, vHIT

1. Introduction

Ménière's disease (MD) is a progressive inner ear disorder that affects at least 0.2% of the population in EUA [1]. The symptoms triad of fluctuating hearing loss, tinnitus, and vertigo was described by Prosper Ménière for more than a century and its pathophysiology is still unknown.

For a long time, it was believed that endolymphatic hydrops would be the histopathological substrate of the disease. The cause of hydrops is still unknown and most of the theories are based on altered endolymph production or reabsorption. The hydrops occurs more often in the cochlea and saccule, followed by the utricle and semicircular channels [2]. Recent studies have indicated that hydrops is a finding of the MD, together with the symptoms, since it

INTECH
open science | open minds

© 2017 The Author(s). Licensee InTech. This chapter is distributed under the terms of the Creative Commons Attribution License (http://creativecommons.org/licenses/by/3.0), which permits unrestricted use, distribution, and reproduction in any medium, provided the original work is properly cited.

alone does not explain all the clinical features, including the progression of hearing loss and the frequency of vertigo attacks [3].

According to the criteria of the Bárány Society, MD is classified as definite or probable. In definite MD, the patient should have had two or more spontaneous episodes of vertigo, each lasting from 20 min to 12 h, documented mild to moderate sensorineural hearing loss, aural symptoms (hearing, tinnitus, and fullness) in the affected ear, and exclusion of other vestibular disorders that explain the symptoms. In probable MD, the patient should have had two or more episodes of vertigo or loss of balance, each lasting from 20 min to 24 h, floating aural symptoms (hearing, tinnitus, or fullness) in that ear, and exclusion of other vestibular disorders that explain the symptoms [4].

MD has a fluctuating course and in many cases difficult in clinical management. Progressive hearing loss becomes more frequent and intense dizzying seizures as the disease progresses. All of this increases the challenges of accurate identification, and has probably led to the trial of several tests for identifying MD. The tests are useful tools to assist the otolaryngologist both in diagnosis and prognosis of MD. Identify the site of hydrops, even in cases of severe hearing loss and possible involvement of the asymptomatic ear are useful information on disease management.

These tests includes tonal and speech audiometry /impedance, otoacustic emissions (OAE), electrocochleography (EcochG), vestibular evoked myogenic potentials (VEMP), cochlear hydrops analysis masking procedure (CHAMP) and video head impulse test (vHIT).

2. Electrophysiology

2.1. Tonal and speech audiometry/Impedance

Audiometry is helpful to confirm the diagnosis and it is a part of the criteria of the Bárány Society. In the early stages of the disease, there is a low frequency sensorineural hearing loss that fluctuates in time. In some cases, it also affects high frequency, setting the pattern of inverted U. In later stages, the hearing loss would increase and the audiogram would become more and more flat. Sometimes, a decreased speech discrimination is also mentioned as a common symptom of MD [5]. Hearing loss initially resolves after attacks, but with the disease progression, patients may experience loss of auditory nerve fibers. The impedance is helpful to exclude middle ear pathology.

2.2. Otoacoustic emission (OAE)

Otoacoustic emissions are subliminal sounds detected in the external auditory canal and generated by the outer hair cells. They are useful in the diagnosis of many cochleopathies, including MD.

Authors believe that hydrops causes changes in the hydrodynamic and cochlear biomechanical micromechanism, due to changes in the interciliary bridges caused by the distension of membranes and cells within the cochlear duct. These changes could affect the transmission of the stimulus by outer hair cells, but not necessarily loss of them. The selective atrophy of the short and medium stereocilia at the cochlea's apex is correlated with the hearing loss in low frequencies that occur in the early phase of MD. The OEA can reveal early lesions due to alterations of the cochlear micromechanism not correlated with the auditory thresholds detected in tone audiometry [6].

The distortion product otoacoustic emission (DPOAE) was considered more appropriate than transient otoacoustic emission (TEOAE) for monitoring during glycerol test because of its high sensitivity in the detection of changes in cochlear function. DPOAE is a complementary test to pure tone audiometry during the glycerol test. It is very useful and will improve the diagnosis of endolymphatic hydrops [7].

2.3. Electrocochleography (EcochG)

Electrocochleography records the three mechanoelectrical potentials of the cochlea. The cochlear microphonic is considered the first step to the neural impulse. It reflects the sum of the intracellular potentials generated in the hair cells of the basal portion of the cochlea during depolarization [8]. Hall in 2007, Durrant, Ding and Salvi in 1998, affirm that the inner hair cells play a central role in the generation of SP, while other authors, such as Burkand et al. believe that it is generated by both internal and external hair cell [8–10]. Action potential (AP) is the sum of the synchrony of individual neural APs of the cochlear nerve.

Electrocochleography is the test capable of measuring endolymphatic hydrops in the cochlea. The test is usually performed with a transthympanic or extrathympanic electrode (**Figure 1**). Hydrops changes the mechanical properties of the cochlea, leading to asymmetric movements of the basilar membrane, which may exacerbate the SP, and consequently, increases the ratio between the amplitudes of SP and AP. The increase in SP amplitude will change according to the existing pressure and volume of the intralabirintic fluid [10, 11] (**Figure 2**).

The SP/AP ratio thresholds are variable in the literature. Pappas et al. believe that any result above 0.5 in an extratympanic EcochG is suggestive of endolymphatic hydrops [12], while Iseli and Gibson established a value of 0.33 in a transtympanic EcoghG [13].

Lamounier et al. in a systematic review reported that in 25–54% of patients with MD, the electrocochleography presented normal results, with the sensitive of the test ranging from 57 to 71% and a specificity ranging from 92 to 96%. In most studies selected, the transtympanic electrode is the most widely used. EcochG in MD presents a variable sensitivity, as in cases of hearing loss due to disease progression, patients may experience a reduction in the amplitude of AP due to loss of auditory nerve fibers [14–17].

On comparing the results of the transtympanic and extratympanic electrocochleography in 20 patients with Ménière's disease and 20 control patients, Ghosh et al. reported a significant difference between the SP/AP ratios of the cases and control groups. For an SP/AP ratio of 0.29, they found 100% sensitivity, 90% specificity to transtympanic, and 90% and 80% to the extratympanic EcochG, respectively, and concluded that extratympanic EcochG is a non-invasive method, effective and easier to carry out in clinical practice than transtympanic EcochG [15].

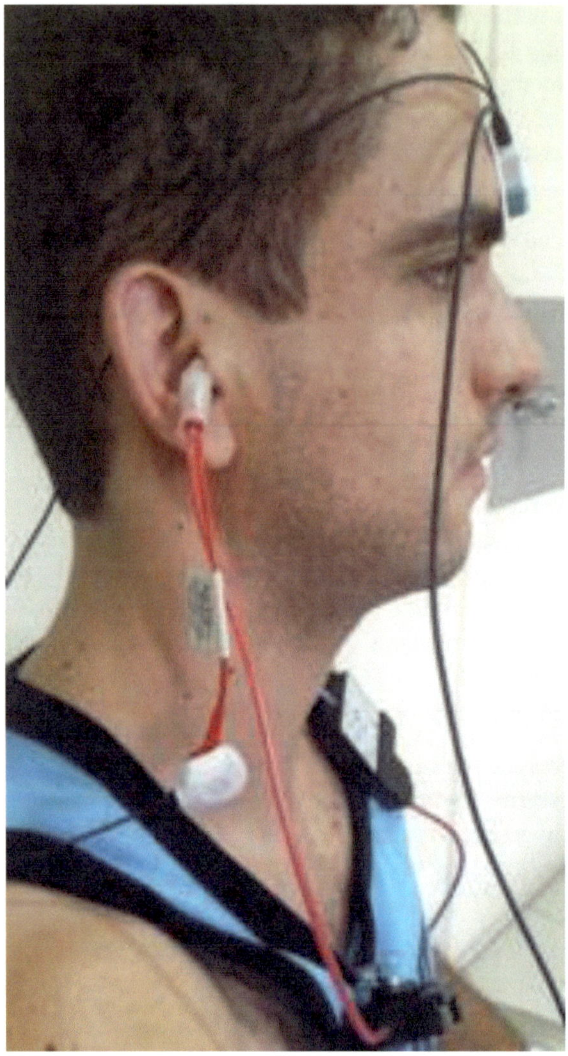

Figure 1. Position of EcochG´s electrodes.

Lamounier et al. also found in the systematic review that the analysis of the SP/AP ratio curve of the transtympanic electrocochleography did not necessarily increase sensitivity in the diagnosis of hydrops when compared with the SP/AP amplitude [14, 16–18].

Gibson et al. compared EcochG results in ears with Ménière's disease and healthy ears with similar hearing loss and concluded that click SP/AP measurements are not helpful in making this differentiation but that tone burst SP amplitude measurements were significantly different between these populations [19].

Colon and Gibson showed that the sensitivity of transtympanic electrocochleography increased to 85% when 1 kHz of tone burst was used to measure SP. They reported that the majority of

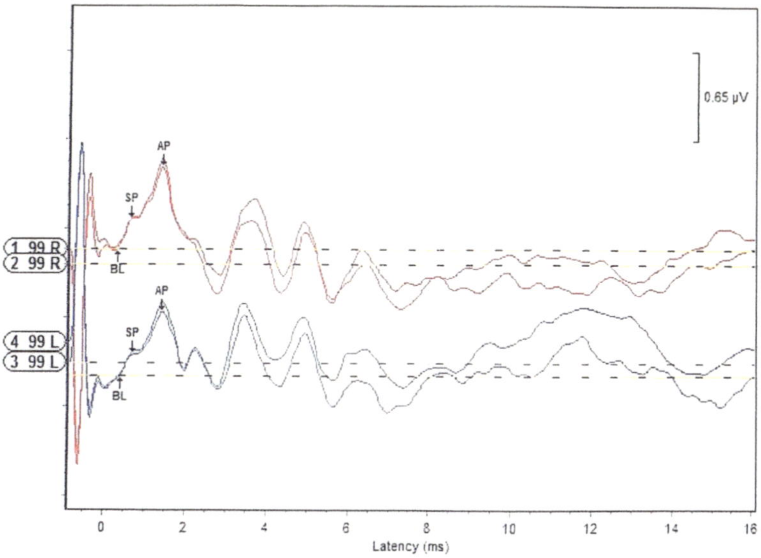

Figure 2. EcochG.

specialists or 58.6%, use click stimuli as opposed to 17.2%, who use tone burst, and 24.3% who use both stimuli [20]. Lopes et al. evaluated the sensitivity and specificity of the SP/AP ratio and graphic angular measurement in electrocochleographies of 71 ears of 41 MD patients and 14 normal-hearing control patients. They concluded that the graphic angular measurement is not sensitive or specific enough to diagnose MD. The association of the SP/AP ratio and graphic angular measurement in conjunction improved the sensitivity to the detriment of the specificity of the test [21].

Electrocochleography is a valuable tool in the diagnosis of cochlear hydrops, as it is noninvasive, easy to handle, and offers new techniques to increase the sensitivity of the test.

2.4. Vestibular evoked myogenic potentials (VEMP)

Vestibular evoked myogenic potentials (VEMP) emerged as a recent and complementary way of vestibular system assessment with the specific analysis of the saccular function and inferior vestibular nerve.

In 1992, Colebatch and Halmagyi proposed that the saccular macula was the peripheral receptor of the vestibular-spinal reflex and in 1994 reported surface potential in the sternocleidomastoid (SCM) muscle in response to clicks through high-intensity air conduction (100 dB), accessing the Sacculo-collic reflex [22].

VEMP is, therefore, a short latency myogenic response, generated after a sound stimulus, originating in the sacculo and conducted by the inferior division of the inferior vestibular nerve to the central nervous system, generating inhibitory electrical responses captured by surface electrodes on the muscles, during muscular contraction. This neural response is a reflex arc of three neurons that surround the inner ear, the brainstem, and the vestibular-spinal pathway [22–24] (**Figure 3**).

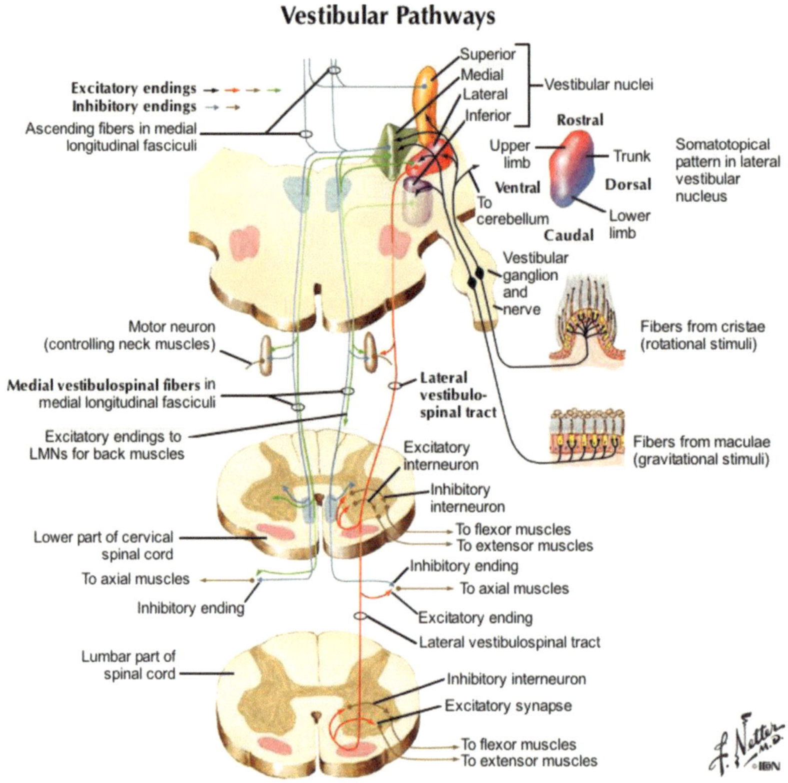

Figure 3. Neural pathway of VEMP.

Similar myogenic responses have been captured in other muscle groups. The responses captured in SCM are called cervical VEMP (cVEMP) and those collected in the extraocular musculature are called ocular VEMP (oVEMP). VEMP can be obtained by air and bone conduction and galvanic stimulation, using tone burst or clicks stimulus [23–25] (**Figure 4**).

The electrical responses of these potentials consist of two biphasic waves, the first negative wave, with latency around 13 ms, known as p13. This is followed by another wave, this time positive, with latency around 23 ms, known as n23. There is also a second biphasic complex known as n34-p44, but due to the lack of replicability of this second complex, only the first complex is considered. The electromyographic potential recording waves are usually defined by: latency, wave morphology, peak-to-peak amplitude, or the difference in values between the most positive point of one wave and the most negative point of another wave [26] (**Figure 5**).

The large variation in the amplitude of the responses, due to the different degrees of muscular contracture obtained for each individual, justifies the analysis of the VEMP responses through the interaural asymmetry index. The literature review showed that VEMP is considered altered by the absence of reproducible waves and or asymmetry index of interaural responses greater than 34% [26].

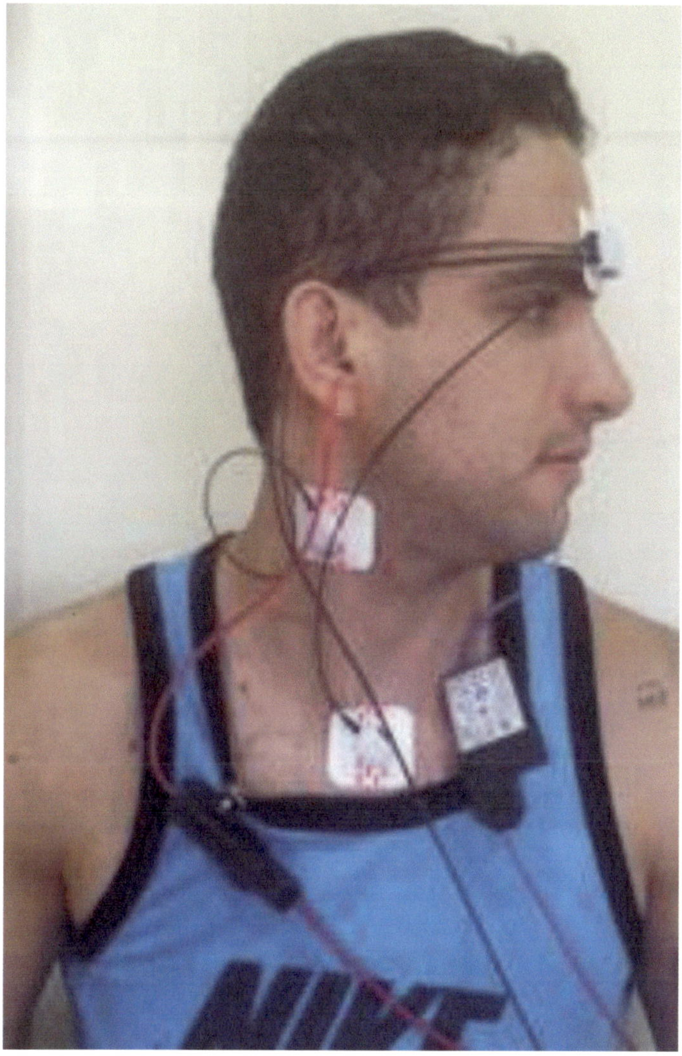

Figure 4. Position of cervical VEMP's electrodes.

The cVEMP is more sensitive for deep bass. Stimuli with frequencies near 500 Hz have higher response amplitudes. Air conducted (AC) sound is the most commonly used stimulus for eliciting cVEMPs. Tone bursts are preferable above clicks because the latter have less reliable results and need higher absolute intensities to evoke a response [26].

The cVEMP is absent or decreased by 30–54% in patients with MD [22, 23]. It may be increased in the early stages of MD, perhaps by the pressure of saccular hydrops against the stapes footplate, increasing sensitivity sacular to intense sound. Its measurement may be floating, with a tendency to disappear with the progression of the disease, as well as 24 h post-crisis, which may reappear after 48 h or with the use of drugs to reduce endolymphatic hydrops [25–27].

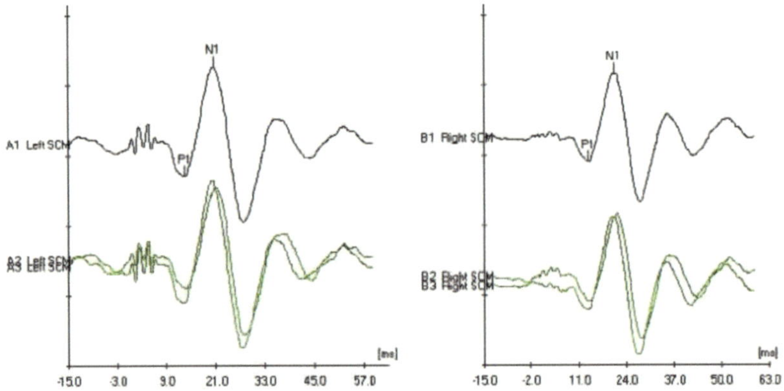

Figure 5. VEMP ´s waves.

Lamounier et al. evaluated the sensitivity and specificity of VEMP and EcochG in the diagnosis of definite MD compared with the clinical diagnosis. The study includes 12 patients (24 ears) diagnosed with definite MD defined according to the clinical criteria proposed by the American Academy of Otolaryngology Head and Neck Surgery (AAO-HNS) in 1995, as well as 12 healthy volunteers allocated to the control group (24 ears). A clinical diagnosis by the AAO-HNS criteria was considered as the gold standard. All patients underwent an otoneurological examination, including pure tone and speech audiometry, cVEMP and extratympanic EcochG. The sensitivity and specificity to detect the presence or absence of disease were calculated. In both tests and in both ears, the ability to diagnose healthy cases was high, with specificity ranging from 84.6 to 100%. Moreover, the ability of the tests to diagnose the disease varied from low to moderate sensitivity, with values ranging from 37.5 to 63.6%. The agreement of both tests in the right ear, measured by the kappa coefficient, was equal to 0.54 indicating a moderate agreement. In the left ear, that agreement was equal to 0.07 indicating a weak correlation between the tests. The sensitivity of the VEMP for the right ear was 63.6% and for the left ear, 62.5%. The sensitivity of EcochG for the right ear was 63.6% and 37.5% for the left ear. They concluded that the specificity of both tests was high, and the sensitivity of VEMP was higher than that of EcochG [3].

Similar to cVEMPs, oVEMPs can also be augmented in MD [28].

The ocular VEMP (oVEMP) is a more recently described reflex, which is thought to reflect predominantly utricular otolith function and can be understood as part of the vestibulo-ocular reflex (VOR). Patients with MD have higher rates of attenuated or absent oVEMPs than normal subjects, increasing with advancing disease [28–30].

Wen et al. recruited unilateral MD patients with either augmented or reduced oVEMPs (asymmetry >40 and <100%) in response to bone-conducted vibration and found that augmented oVEMPs were seen more frequently in patients with early stage MD. Augmented responses might also be more likely when recorded during an attack [31].

Winters et al. examined air-conducted oVEMPs in MD patients and found lower response rates with smaller amplitudes and higher thresholds compared to normal subjects. Interestingly, this effect was observed not only in the affected, but to a lesser extent also in the clinically unaffected ears [32].

The VEMP is easy to perform, does not cause discomfort to patient and does not vary with hearing loss. The ability to predict the presence of abnormalities in an asymptomatic ear is one of the great features of VEMP [33].

2.5. Cochlear hydrops analysis masking procedure (CHAMP)

The cochlear hydrops analysis masking procedure (CHAMP) was introduced in 2005 as a new test to diagnose MD. Don et al. showed that endolymphatic hydrops in patients diagnosed with MD causes changes in the response properties of the basilar membrane that lead to impaired high-pass noise masking of auditory brainstem response (ABR) to clicks in staked ABR. The latency delay in normal-hearing ears, between wave V for the click alone response and the 0.5 kHz high-pass masking noise condition, is significantly longer than that in MD ears. This difference is known as the latency delay [34].

The increased velocity of the traveling wave would affect the properties of the basilar membrane but cannot affect the tonotopic organization along the basilar membrane. The increased velocity of the traveling wave is more likely to impact the low frequencies as they are represented toward the apical end on the basilar membrane. When ABR latencies are obtained by presenting clicks along with the high-pass masking noise in individuals with Méniére's disease, the altered motion mechanics of the basilar membrane limits the ability of low-frequency noise to mask the activity in high frequency [35, 36] (**Figure 6**).

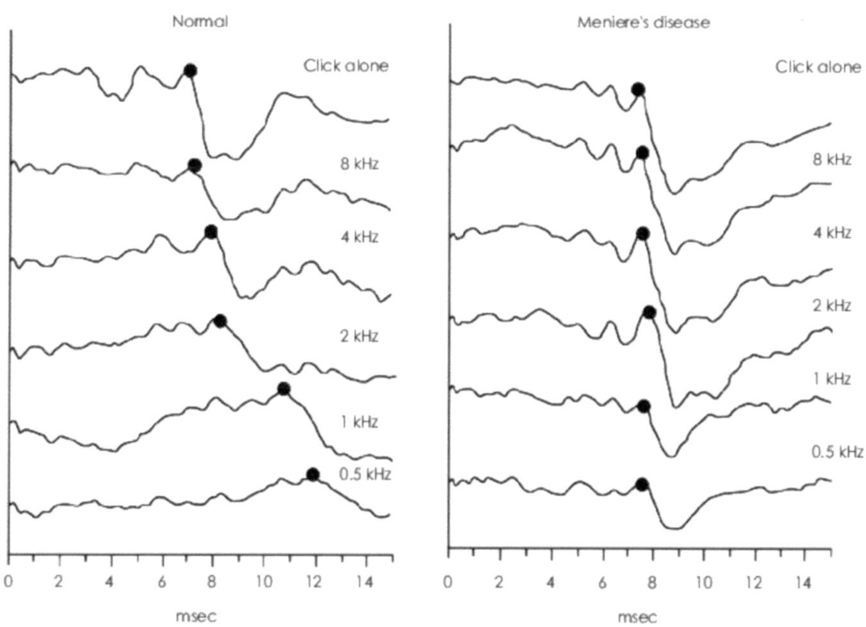

Figure 6. CHAMP.

In individuals with MD, we can observe the phenomenon of undermasking in high-pass responses, whereas the undermasking phenomenon is not seen in normal individuals. This would in turn result in lesser latency difference between click alone and click with 500 Hz high-pass masking noise condition in ears with MD than unaffected or normal ears [37].

Don et al. conducted the test in 23 definite MD patients and compared the results with 38 non-MD normal-hearing subjects. Their measures did not demonstrate an overlap between the Ménière's and nonMénière's groups, and therefore, the authors concluded that the test had an extremely high, even 100%, sensitivity and 100% specificity for diagnostic use in individual patients [34].

However, some studies have questioned these findings by reporting significantly lower sensitivity and specificity values. De Valck et al. evaluated CHAMP performance in Ménière patients and normal controls, and revealed no discriminative value in differentiating Ménière's from non-MD subjects with otovestibular symptoms [37].

Kingma investigated the usefulness of the cochlear hydrops analysis masking procedure (CHAMP) as an additional diagnostic test in patients with definite unilateral Ménière's disease. With less than 0.3 ms criterion and including the ears in which no delay could be measured, the sensitivity of the CHAMP is 32% and concluded that abnormal latency delays for CHAMP are delays shorter than 2 ms. Earlier results with CHAMP should be reconsidered using this criterion, instead of 0.3 ms [38].

Lee et al. suggest that the CHAMP seems to be more valuable in detection of definite MD than is extratympanic EcochG [39].

Furthermore, CHAMP can only be recorded for losses not exceeding moderate degree, which limits its use to identify Meniere's disease with lesser degree of hearing losses only.

The literature indicates a need for continued exploration of these tests in order to establish the usefulness or lack of it in the diagnosis for MD.

2.6. Video head impulse test (vHIT)

A new quantitative test of vestibular function known as the video head impulse test (vHIT) has recently emerged that now allows for discrete measurements of the vestibulo-ocular reflex (VOR) during evaluation of the extremely high-frequency head movements. Although the bithermal caloric test is useful for assessing low-frequency vestibular system function, the head impulse test (HIT), as described by Halmagyi and Curthoys, is a method for testing the function in a frequency region encountered in everyday life in the vestibular system [40, 41].

The primary differences between the vHIT and caloric tests are the mode of stimulus delivery (thermal gradient vs. natural head motion) as well as the temporal frequency of each examination (caloric stimulus represents a low-frequency stimulus and the vHIT a high-frequency stimulus). It is well known that the vHIT and caloric tests are sensitive to detection of a certain percentage of patients with MD [42, 43].

The test involves examiner-initiated high velocity, high-acceleration, and yet, small-amplitude head movements while the patient is instructed to stare at a stationary target located at center gaze. If the VOR is intact, the patient will be able to maintain foveal vision of the target during the head impulse. If the VOR is impaired, rotation of the head toward the ipsilesional semicircular canal will drive the eyes off the target, forcing the patient to generate a volitional catch-up saccade to bring eyes back to the target [40] (**Figures 7** and **8**).

The receptor of the angular VOR is the crista ampullaris. This structure consists of both type I and type II hair cells as well as regularly and irregularly discharging afferent neurons. Type I hair cells populate the central part of the crista ampullaris. Irregular afferents primarily connect to type I hair cells or a mixture of type I and type II. These hair cells encode high-frequency, high-acceleration head movements. Type II cells populate the periphery of the crista. Regular afferents carry the output of type II hair cells or a mixture of type I and type II and likely encode low-frequency, low acceleration movement [44, 45].

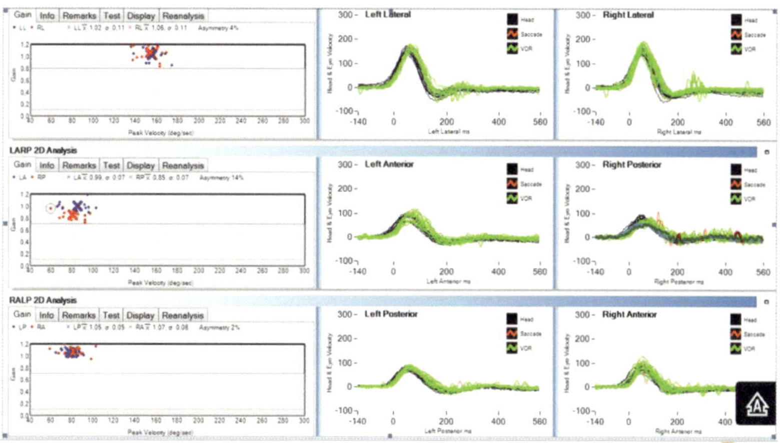

Figure 7. VHIT : Speed of the head in black = speed the eyes in green. There is no record of corrective saccades. (Figure provided by borgesdecarvalhootorrinos.com.br).

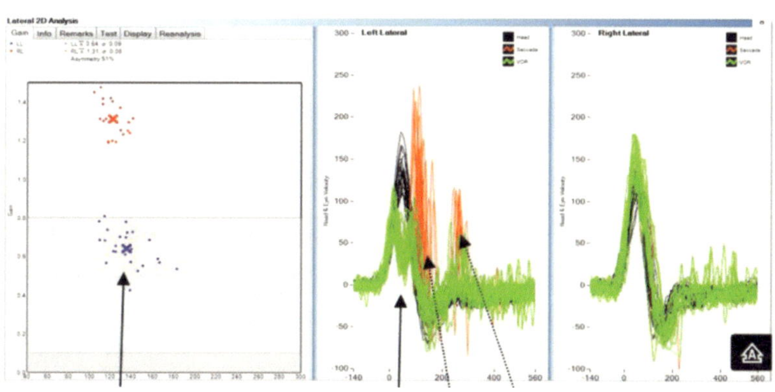

Figure 8. VHIT: Lower eye velocity than head. Presence of saccades. (Figure provided by borgesdecarvalhootorrinos.com.br).

Tsuji et al. reported that although MD affected the structure and function of type II hair cells, the density and number of type I hair cells appeared unchanged in patients with MD [46].

Maire and van Melle showed that, in early stages of MD, VOR gain was higher when the patient was rotated toward the affected ear, but this observed enhancement diminished as the disease progressed [47].

McCaslin et al. presented three cases of patients with Ménière's disease with asymptomatic vestibular dysfunction demonstrated with videonystagmography (VNG) testing, which provided a quantitative measure of VOR gain. The authors found a dissociation between the caloric test and VHIT results, and they explained these findings by understanding the different dynamic response properties of the two primary populations of neurons in the crista [40].

The assessment of cochlear function with audiometry, EcochG and CHAMP, of the saccule through cervical VEMP, of the utricle through ocular VEMP, of the lateral semicircular canal with the caloric tests, and all of the semicircular canals by the vHIT demonstrates the advancements of research in the vestibular diagnosis. New paths are open to the discovery of the pathophysiological mechanism of a disease that was first described over a century ago and still has no defined treatment protocol.

Author details

Pauliana Lamounier

Address all correspondence to: paulilamounier@yahoo.com.br

Centro de Reabilitação e Readaptação Dr Henrique Santillo—CRER, Goiânia, GO, Brazil

References

[1] Lacour M, van de Heyning PH, Novotny M, Brahim T. Betahistine in the treatment of Ménière's disease. Neuropsychiatric Disease and Treatment. 2007;**3**(4):429-440

[2] Okuno T, Sando I. Localization, frequency and severity of endolymphatic hydrops and the pathology of the labyrinthine membrane in Ménière's disease. The Annals of Otology, Rhinology, and Laryngology. 1987;**96**:438-445

[3] Lamounier P, de Souza TSA, Gobbo DA, Bahmad Jr. F. Evaluation of vestibular evoked myogenic potentials (VEMP) and electrocochleography for the diagnosis of Ménière's disease. Brazilian Journal of Otorhinolaryngology. 2016. DOI: 10.1016/j.bjorl.2016.04.021

[4] Escamez JAL, Carey J, Chung WH, Goebel JA, Magnusson M, Mandala M, et al. Diagnostic criteria for Menière's disease. Consensus document of the Bárány Society, The Japan Society for Equilibrium Research, the European Academy of Otology and Neurotology (EAONO), the American Academy of Otolaryngology-Head and Neck

Surgery (AAO-HNS) and theKorean Balance Society. Acta Otorrinolaringológica Española. 2016;**67**(1):1-7

[5] Mateijsen DJM, Van Hengel PWJ, Van Huffelen WM, Wit HP, Albers FWJ. Pure-tone and speech audiometry in patients with Meniere's disease. Clinical Otolaryngology. 2001;**26**:379-387

[6] Aquino AMCM, Massaro CAM, Tiradentes JB, Garzon JCV, Oliveira JAA. Otoacoustic emissions in early diagnosis of cochlear lesions in Méniére's disease. Revista Brasileira de Otorrinolaringologia. 2002;**68**(5):761-765

[7] Sakashita T, Kubo T, Kyunai K, Ueno K, Hikawa C, et al. Changes in otoacoustic emission during the glycerol test in the ears of patients with Ménière's disease. Nihon Jibiinkoka Gakkai Kaiho. 2001;**104**(6):682-693

[8] Burkard RF, Eggermont JJ, Don M. Auditory evoked potentials: Basic principles and clinical application. In: Electric and Magnetic Fields of Synchronous Neural Activity. Baltimore: Lippincott Williams & Wilkins; 2007. pp.2-21

[9] Hall JW, Antonelli PJ. Assessment of peripheral and central auditory function. In: Bailey BJ, Jackler RK, Pillsbury HC 3rd, Lambert PR, editors. Head and Neck Surgery-Otolaryngology. 3rd ed. Lippincott, Philadelphia: Williams and Wilkins; 2001. p. 1666

[10] Durrant J, Wang J, Ding D, Salvi R. Are inner or outer hair cells the source of summating potentials recorded from the round window? Journal of the Acoustical Society of America. 1998;**104**:370-377

[11] Nguyen LT, Harris JP, Nguyen QT. Clinical utility of electrocochleography in the diagnosis and management of Ménière's disease: AOS and ANS member ship survey data. Otology & Neurotology. 2010;**31**:455-459

[12] Pappas DGJ, Pappas DGS, Carmichael L, Hyatt DP, Toohey LM. Extratympanic electrocochleography: Diagnostic and predictive value. American Journal of Otolaryngology. 2000;**21**:81-87

[13] Iseli C, Gibson WA. Comparison of three methods of using transtympanic electrocochleography for the diagnosis of Ménière's disease: Click summating potential measurements, tone burst summating potential amplitude measurements, and biasing of the summating potential using a low frequency tone. Acta Oto-Laryngologica. 2010;**130**:95-101

[14] Lamounier P, Gobbo DA, de Souza TS, de Oliveira CA, Bahmad F Jr. Electrocochleography for Ménière's disease: Is it reliable? Brazilian Journal of Otorhinolaryngology. 2014; **80**:527-532

[15] Ghosh S, Gupta AK, Mann SS. Can electrocochleography in Meniere's disease be noninvasive? The Journal of Otolaryngology. 2002;**31**:371-375

[16] Baba A, Takasaki K, Tanaka F, Tsukasaki N, Kumagami H, Takahashi H. Amplitude and area ratios of summating potential/action potential (SP/AP) in Ménière's disease. Acta Oto-Laryngologica. 2009;**129**:25-29

[17] Chung WH, Cho DY, Choi JY, Hong SH. Clinical usefulness of extratympanic electrocochleography in the diagnosis of Ménière's disease. Otology & Neurotology. 2004;**25**: 144-149

[18] Devaiah AK, Dawson KL, Ferraro JA, Ator GA. Utility of area curve ratio electrocochleography in early Meniere disease. Archives of Otolaryngology–Head and Neck Surgery. 2003;**129**:547-551

[19] Gibson WP. A comparison of two methods of using transtympanic electrocochleography for the diagnosis of Meniere's disease: Click summating potential/action potential ratio measurements and toneburst summating potential measurements. Acta Oto-Laryngologica. 2009. Suppl;38-42

[20] Conlon BJ, Gibson WP. Electrocochleography in the diagnosis of Meniere's disease. Acta Oto-Laryngologica. 2000;**120**:480-483

[21] Lopes KC, Munhoz MSL, Santos MAR, Moraes MFD, Chaves AG. A medida angular gráfica como parâmetro de avaliação da eletrococleografia. Brazilian Journal of Otorhinolaryngology. 2011;**77**(2):214-220

[22] Rosengren SM, Welgampola MS, Colebatch JG. Vestibular evoked myogenic potentials: Past, present and future. Clinical Neurophysiology. 2010;**121**:636-651

[23] Egami N, Ushio M, Yamasoba T, Yamaguchi T, Murofushi T,Iwasaki S. The diagnostic value of vestibular evoked myogenic potentials in patients with Ménière's disease. Journal of Vestibular Research. 2013;**23**:249-257

[24] Ribeiro S, Almeida RR, Caovilla HH, Ganança MM. Dos potenciais evocados miogênicos vestibulares nas orelhas comprometida e assintomática na Doença de Ménière unilateral. Revista Brasileria Otorrinolaringologia. 2005;**71**:60-66

[25] Young YH, Huang TW, Cheng PW. Assessing the stage of Ménière's disease using vestibular evoked myogenic potentials. Archives of Otolaryngology–Head and Neck Surgery. 2003;**129**:815-818

[26] Duarte PLS. Avaliação dos Potenciais Evocados Miogênicos Vestibulares e Eletrococleografia no diagnóstico da Doença de Ménière. Brasília: Universidade de Brasília; 2015

[27] Kuo SW, Yang TH, Young YH. Changes in vestibular evoked myogenic potentials after Meniere attacks. The Annals of Otology, Rhinology, and Laryngology. 2005;**114**(9):717-721

[28] Weber KP, Rosengren SM. Clinical utility of ocular vestibular-evoked myogenic potentials (oVEMPs). Current Neurology and Neuroscience Reports. 2015;**15**:22

[29] Huang CH, Wang SJ, Young YH. Localization and prevalence of hydrops formation in Meniere's disease using a test battery. Audiology & Neuro-Otology. 2011;**16**(1):41-48

[30] Taylor RL, Wijewardene AA, Gibson WP, Black DA, Halmagyi GM, Welgampola MS. The vestibular evoked-potential profile of Meniere's disease. Clinical Neurophysiology: Official Journal of the International Federation of Clinical Neurophysiology. 2011;**122**(6): 1256-1263

[31] Wen MH, Cheng PW, Young YH. Augmentation of ocular vestibular-evoked myogenic potentials via bone-conducted vibration stimuli in Meniere disease. Otolaryngology–Head and Neck Surgery: Official Journal of American Academy of Otolaryngology–Head and Neck Surgery. 2012;**146**(5):797-803

[32] Winters SM, Campschroer T, Grolman W, Klis SF. Ocular vestibular evoked myogenic potentials in response to air-conducted sound in Meniere's disease. Otolaryngology–Head and Neck Surgery: Official Journal of American Academy of Otolaryngology–Head and Neck Surgery. 2011;**32**(8):1273-1280

[33] Adams ME, Heidenreich KD, Kileny PR. Audiovestibular testing in patients with Ménière's disease. Otolaryngologic Clinics of North America 2010;**43**:995-1009

[34] Don M, Kwong B, Tanaka C. A diagnostic test for Meniere's disease and cochlear hydrops: Impaired high-pass noise masking of auditory brainstem response. Otology & Neurotology. 2005;**26**(4):711-722

[35] Donaldson GS, Ruth RA. Derived-band auditory brainstem response estimates of traveling wave velocity in humans: II. Subjects with noise-induced hearing loss and Meniere's disease. Journal of Speech, Language, and Hearing Research. 1996;**39**(3):534-545

[36] Singh NK, Krishnamurthy R, Premkumar PK. Relative efficiency of cochlear hydrops analysis masking procedure and cervical vestibular evoked myogenic potential in identification of Meniere's disease. Advances in Otolaryngology. 2015. DOI: 10.1155/2015/978161

[37] De Valck CFJ, Claes GME, Wuyts FL, Van de Heyning PH. Lack of diagnostic value of high-pass noise masking of auditory brainstem responses in Ménière's disease. Otology & Neurotology. 2007;**28**:700-707

[38] Kingma CM, Wit HP. Cochlear hydrops analysis masking procedure results in patients with unilateral Ménière's disease. Otology & Neurotology. 2010;**31**(6):1004-1008

[39] Lee JB, et al. Diagnostic efficiency of the cochlear hydrops analysis masking procedure in Meniere's disease. Otology & Neurotology. 2011;**32**:1486-1491

[40] McCaslin DL, Rivas A, Jacobson GP, Bennett ML. The dissociation of video head impulse test (Vhit) and bithermal caloric test results provide topological localization of vestibular system impairment in patients with "Definite" Ménière's disease. American Journal of Audiology. 2015;**24**:1-10

[41] Halmagyi GM, Curthoys IS. A clinical sign of canal paresis. Archives of Neurology. 1988 Jul;**45**(7):737-739

[42] McCaslin DL, Jacobson GP. Current role of the videonystagmography examination in the context of the multidimensional balance function test battery. Seminars in Hearing. 2009;**30**(4):242-252

[43] McCaslin DL, Jacobson GP, Bennett ML, Gruenwald JM, Green AP. Predictive properties of the video head impulse test: Measures of caloric symmetry and self-report dizziness handicap. Ear and Hearing. 2014;**35**(5):185-191

[44] Hullar TE, Della Santina CC, Hirvonen T, Lasker DM, Carey JP, Minor LB. Responses of irregularly discharging chinchilla semicircular canal vestibular-nerve afferents during high-frequency head rotations. Journal of Neurophysiology. 2005;**93**(5):2777-2786

[45] Hullar TE, Minor LB. High-frequency dynamics of regularly discharging canal afferents provide a linear signal for angular vestibuloocular reflexes. Journal of Neurophysiology. 1999 Oct;**82**(4):2000-2005

[46] Tsuji K, Velázquez-Villaseñor L, Rauch SD, Glynn RJ, Wall C 3rd, Merchant SN. Temporal bone studies of the human peripheral vestibular system. Meniere's disease. The Annals of Otology, Rhinology, and Laryngology. Suppl. 2000 May;**181**:26-31

[47] Maire R, van Melle G. Vestibulo-ocular reflex characteristics in patients with unilateral Ménière's disease. Otology & Neurotology. 2008 Aug;**29**(5):693-698

Chapter 8

Hearing and Vestibular Testing in Menière's Disease

Madalina Gabriela Georgescu

Additional information is available at the end of the chapter

http://dx.doi.org/10.5772/66382

Abstract

Audiological and vestibular testing plays an important role in diagnosis of Menière's disease,as disease *per se* and as staging diagnosis. A battery of tests are recommended in order to have a better evaluation of the disease. Audiological testing includes pure tone audiometry, with highlights of bone conduction especially in acute episodes of Menière's disease, speech audiometry and glycerol test when hearing loss is documented, ABR and electrocochleography. Besides these investigations, vestibular investigations are also recommended in order to evaluate the degree of vestibular lesion present from the beginning of Menière's disease—electro- and videonystagmography, head impulse test, vestibular evoked myogenic potentials and computerized dynamic posturography.

Keywords: pure tone audiometry, glycerol test, auditory brainstem response, vestibular evoked myogenic potentials

1. Introduction

The aim of this chapter is to clearly identify the usefulness of audiological investigations, both for hearing and for vestibular function, in positive diagnosis of Menière's disease and in staging the lesion. This is important for counselling the patients regarding the disease long-term evolution and also for appropriate management of the disease.

Inner ear spaces of the anterior and posterior labyrinth communicate in between and endolymphatic hydrops present in the Menière's disease usually affects both auditory and vestibular sensorial structures located in the two parts of the inner ear.

In this chapter, hearing and vestibular testing will be presented, as tests are recommended for positive and differential diagnosis of the Menière's disease. Regarding Menière's disease diagnostic, audiological and vestibular testing plays an important role in diagnosis of the disease *per se* and for staging diagnosis. Besides medical importance, accurate diagnosis is also

INTECH
open science | open minds

© 2017 The Author(s). Licensee InTech. This chapter is distributed under the terms of the Creative Commons Attribution License (http://creativecommons.org/licenses/by/3.0), which permits unrestricted use, distribution, and reproduction in any medium, provided the original work is properly cited. (cc) BY

important for counselling the patients regarding the disease long-term evolution and also for appropriate management of the disease.

2. Audiological evaluation

Audiological testing includes pure tone audiometry, with highlights of bone conduction especially in acute episodes of this disease, glycerol test when hearing loss is documented, auditory brainstem response (ABR) and electrocochleography.

2.1. Pure tone audiometry

Pure tone audiometry is a subjective method of hearing evaluation. Patient must signalize the faintest sound he/she hears. Pure tone with specific frequencies is used (125, 250, 500, 1000, 2000, 4000, and 8000 Hz), based on the human normal hearing frequency range (20–20,000 Hz).

Sounds are presented both in air and bone conduction in order to have an accurate image of the hearing.

The result of the test is shown in a graph, a Cartesian system with frequency tested (in Hz) on horizontal axis and intensity (in dB HL) on the vertical one. Frequency varies between 125 and 8000 Hz and intensity between −10 and 120 dB (the latest represents the painful sensation, not an audible one = uncomfortable level). Based on patient's response, the least audible intensity (threshold) on each tested frequency is plotted.

Threshold notation is standardized internationally (ISO system) and colors as well: red for the right ear and blue for the left ear (**Figure 1**):

- Air conduction: "circle" for the right ear and "X" for the left ear
- Nose-opened brackets for bone conduction: "<" and ">" in unmasked condition and "[" and "]" in masked condition

Normative for hearing thresholds (THR) were established based on nonotological history teenagers' responses decades ago and normal hearing stands for hearing thresholds between −10 and +20 dB on all frequencies, without differences between air and bone conduction (**Figure 2**).

Pure tone audiometry is the method of choice for hearing evaluation also in Menière's disease patients in [1, 2]. When hearing loss (HL) is permanent, Menière's disease patients experience

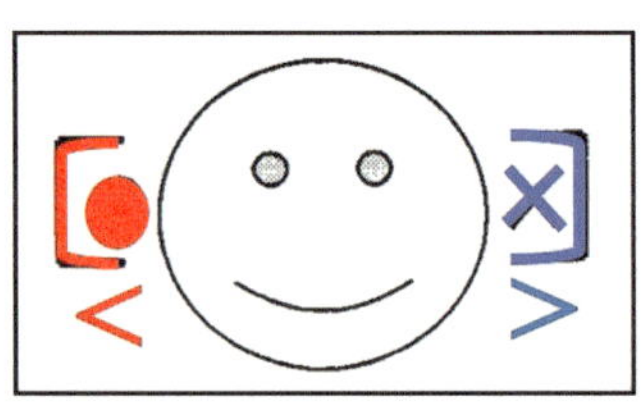

Figure 1. Standardized notation for hearing thresholds.

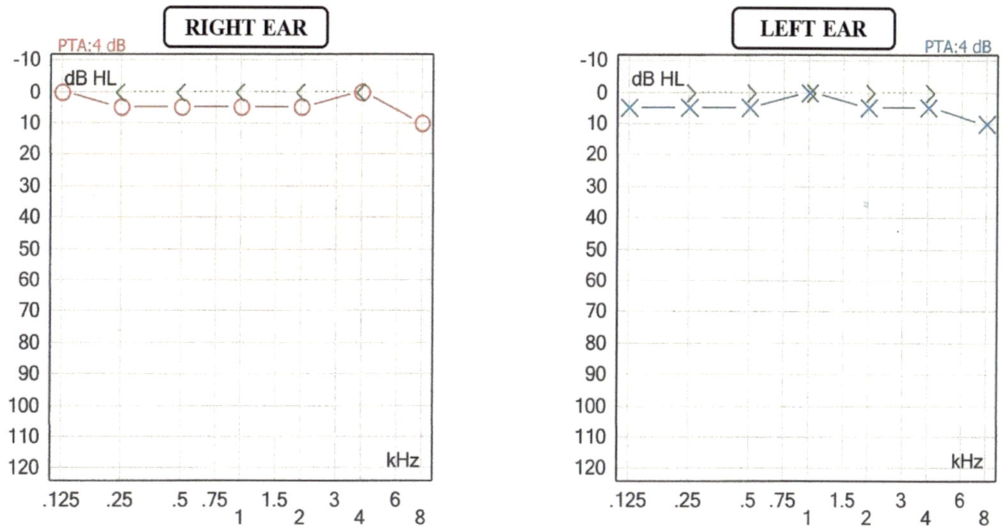

Figure 2. Pure tone audiometry—normal hearing in both ears.

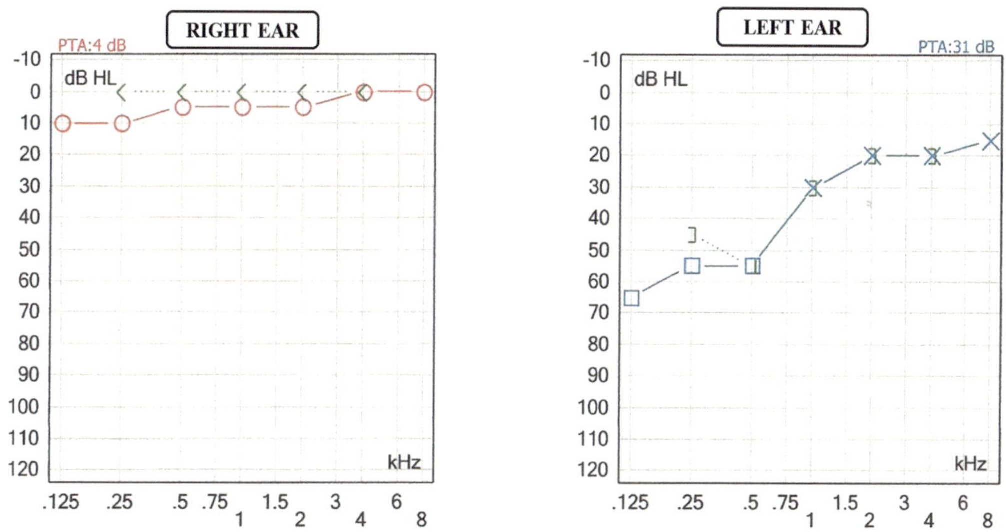

Figure 3. Low frequency sensorineural hearing loss in left ear.

sensorineural hearing loss (average of hearing THR on 0.5, 1, and 2 kHz greater than 20 dB), with pathological thresholds on low frequencies (**Figure 3**).

Cochlear sensorineural hearing loss (SNHL) is accompanied by recruitment, a phenomenon of increased loudness perception—above an increase threshold, higher intensity sounds are as loud to the hearing impaired person as for a normal hearing one and thus disturbing.

Some authors describe in Menière's disease patients a particular type of recruitment—hyper- or overrecruitment: loudness in the affected ear overtakes the normal ear at high intensities in [3–5].

When differences between air conduction thresholds in both ears exceed 40dB for supra-aural earphones or 55 dB when insert earphones are used, air conduction masking is mandatory for that specific frequency where this difference exists. For bone conduction, masking is mandatory whenever more than 10dB difference between bone and air conduction thresholds is present on that specific frequency. Bone conduction masking is essential in differentiating conductive and sensorineural hearing loss.

It is not unusual to have a conductive component of the hearing loss in Menière's disease acute phase—disturbances in endolymph metabolism lead to pressure variations at the round and oval window with secondary increases of impedances. High impedances diminish air transmission of the sounds, with consecutive cochlear conductive hearing loss (**Figure 4**). In these cases, middle ear test (tympanometry and acoustically evoked stapedius reflex) shows no impairment of the middle ear as cause of the conductive component of the hearing loss.

2.2. Speech audiometry

Besides pure tone audiometry, speech audiometry complements auditory evaluation. It is a more complex test, since evaluates the entire auditory pathway as hearing is a cortical process. Speech audiometry is also a subjective audiological test where the tested person has to repeat the heard stimuli—numbers, monosyllabic, disyllabic words, or sentences.

The result of the test is a Cartesian graphic with percentage of correct repeated stimuli on the vertical axis for each intensity tested and with intensity of the stimulus on the horizontal axis. For each intensity, a phonemic-balanced list of 10 stimuli (numbers, monosyllabic, disyllabic words, or sentences) is presented. These percentages draw a curve which crosses the 50% line at some specific intensity. This crossing represents the threshold of speech audiometry. For normal hearing, conductive or cochlear sensorial sensorineural hearing loss, this threshold must correlate with pure tone average ±7 dB (**Figure 5**).

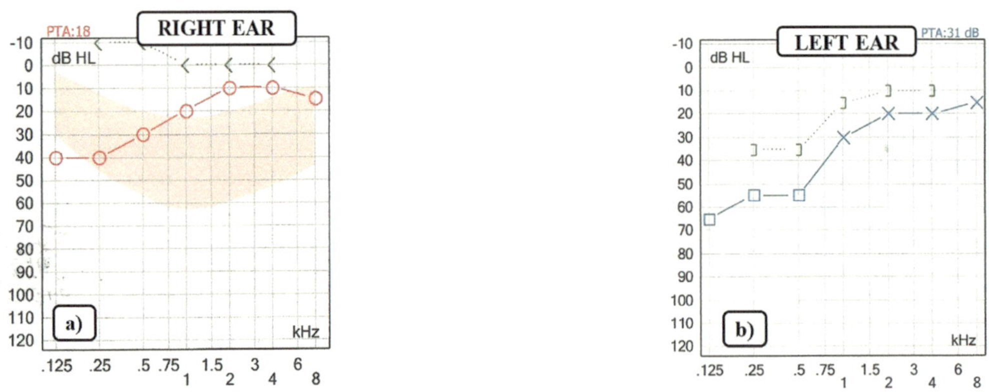

Figure 4. Conductive (a) or mixed (b) hearing loss due to cochlear conductive hearing loss.

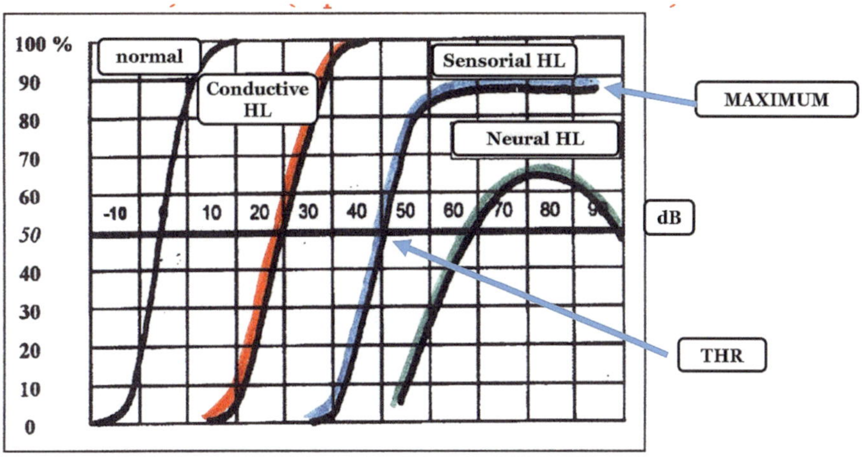

Figure 5. Speech audiometry.

If in cochlear sensorineural hearing loss of other etiology there is a good correlation (±7 dB) between pure tone and speech audiometry THR, in prolonged Menière's disease, some differences may appear.

Another parameter used in interpretation of the speech audiometry is the maxim of intelligibility/discrimination. It represents the highest percentage of correct repeated stimuli the patient obtains. For normal hearing or conductive hearing loss persons, 100% intelligibility is reached.

Sensorineural hearing loss induced distortions in audition which can limit the maximum of discrimination. Speech audiometry can draw attention on the estimated site of hearing loss, cochlear, or retrocochlear: in cochlear lesions, once the maximum score of discrimination is reached, it remains constant as higher intensities are tested. In retrocochlear sensorineural hearing loss an odd phenomenon occurs—as intensity increases, the patient understands less word (roll-over phenomenon).

2.3. Glycerol test

In patients with Menière's disease and permanent sensorineural HL, if low frequencies THR are greater than 40 dB, glycerol test is recommended. Since endolymphatic hydrops is the pathophysiological mechanism of the Menière's disease, oral administration of a hypertonic solution will extract liquids from tissues, including from the endolymphatic space. Thus, the endolymphatic pressure is diminished and hearing and vestibular sensorial epithelium recovers from increased pressure. The clinical effect of this restoration is improvement of both auditory and vestibular system function 2 h and 30 min after the ingestion, when both pure tone audiometry and speech audiometry are repeated.

Hearing improvement can be documented by pure tone audiometry and speech audiometry. An improvement of the THR on at least 10dB on three consecutive frequencies in pure tone audiometry and/or a more than 12% improvement of speech audiometry THR is considered

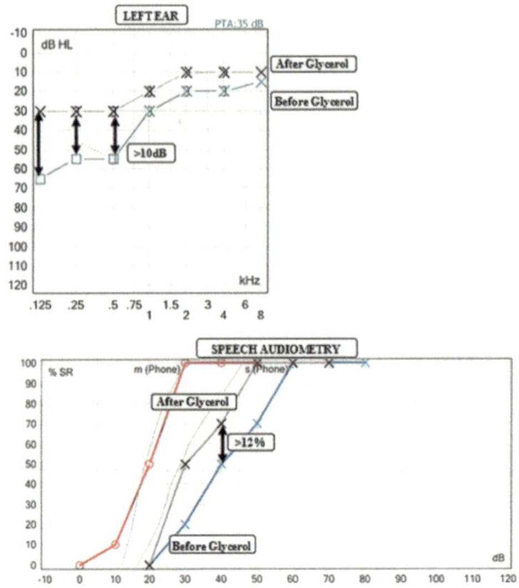

Figure 6. Positive glycerol test.

a positive glycerol test (**Figure 6**). Some authors consider this as an indication for diuretic treatment, since the endolymphatic system has the capacity to modify its pressure after oral administration of a hyperosmolar solution.

2.4. Brainstem evoked response audiometry (BERA)/auditory brainstem response (ABR)

ABR—is an objective electrophysiological audiological method that allows recording of the electrical activity evoked by neural activity in the auditory pathways, from the cochlea to the brainstem (lateral lemniscus) in Refs. [6, 7]. Surface electrodes are used in this far-field technique. Most commonly used acoustic stimulus is the click—a brief (0.1 ms) rectangular stimulus. Click-evoked ABR reflects hearing sensitivity in the frequency range of 1–4 kHz with a high correlation with pure tone audiometry threshold in this frequency domain, especially at 4 kHz where the stimulus' energy is maximum.

ABR is the first evoked potentials, with seven characteristic waves in the first 10 ms after click stimulation at high intensities: 70–90 dB normal hearing level (nHL). These waves were first described by Jewett, as response of different auditory pathway structures after acoustic stimulation:

- wave I: proximal auditory nerve
- wave II: distal auditory nerve
- wave III: cochlear nuclei
- wave IV: superior olivar complex
- wave V: lateral lemniscus

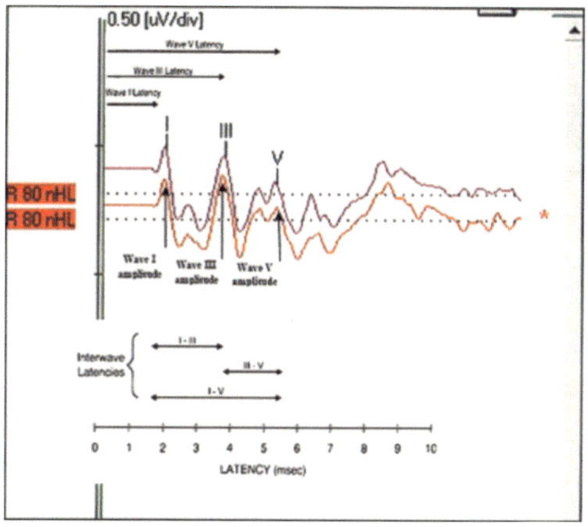

Figure 7. Parameters used in ABR interpretation.

- wave VI: medial geniculate body (thalamus)—probable
- wave VII: medial geniculate body (thalamus)—probable

First five are mostly used in interpretation of the BERA recordings. In Menière's disease patients, BERA is mandatory in order to rule out a retrocochlear etiology of the sensorineural hearing loss. Latencies, interpeak intervals and interaural differences of the latencies and interpeak intervals are the parameters used for this differential diagnosis (**Figure 7**).

In general, ABR exhibits a sensitivity of over 90% and a specificity of approximately 70–90%. Findings suggestive of retrocochlear pathology may include any one or more of the following:

- Absolute latency interaural difference wave V (IT5)—prolonged as compared with normative data.
- I–V interpeak interval interaural difference (IPI1-5)—prolonged as compared with normative data; greater than 0.2 ms in unilateral or symmetrical hearing loss, or greater than 0.3 ms in patients with asymmetrical or with noise-induced hearing loss. Interaural IPI difference criterion requires no correction for audiogram differences.
- Absolute latency of wave V—prolonged as compared with normative data.
- Absolute latencies and interpeak intervals latencies I–III, I–V, III–V—prolonged as compared with normative data.
- Absence of the later waves.
- Absent auditory brainstem response in the involved ear even though hearing is normal or mildly impaired.
- ABR traces not replicable.
- Abnormally low V:I amplitude ratio (less than 1.0)—less sensitivity than latency measurements.

2.5. Electrocochleography

Electrocochleography (ECochG) is an objective audiological test that measures the electrical potentials derived from the cochlear hair cells and the auditory nerve in [8–10]. These potentials are produced between an electrode on the cochlear promontory and an earlobe electrode, within a time frame of 5 ms after stimulation with alternative repetitive very short acoustic signals (click). Averaging of a large number of potentials (1000 sweeps) is needed in order to record the ECochG characteristic wave. Click is the most common stimuli used in ECochG due to its effect of very good synchronization of a large number of cochlear nerve fibers, mandatory for eliciting a measurable action potential. Click has an abrupt onset, very short duration and broad frequency spectra, thus stimulating a very large number of hair cells in the basal turn of the cochlea, where the speed of the travelling wave is the fastest.

Magnitude and quality of the response depends on the electrode type—transtympanic electrode fixed directly on the promontory gives the best recordings, but it is an invasive audiological investigation. Alternatively, with good clinical results are used extratympanic electrodes, place in the external auditory canal, as close as possible to the eardrum or on the eardrum itself.

Synchronization of the auditory nerve fibers after above-mentioned stimulation gives birth to global action potential. Its origin lies into the inner ear hair cells and cochlear nerve.

Global action potential consists of presynaptic and postsynaptic potentials (**Figure 8**).

The first one includes cochlear microphonic (CM) that originates in the outer cochlear hair cells and summating potential (SP) arising from the inner cochlear hair cells. Postsynaptic potentials, known as global action potential of the cochlear nerve, is generated by all cochlear nerve fibers, fired in synchrony by the acoustic stimulus.

In endolymphatic hydrops, due to the increased pressure in scala media, basilar membrane vibrates asymmetrical. These changes of the traveling wave lead to several dysfunctions: distorted cochlear microphonics, enlargement of the summating potential and broadening of the

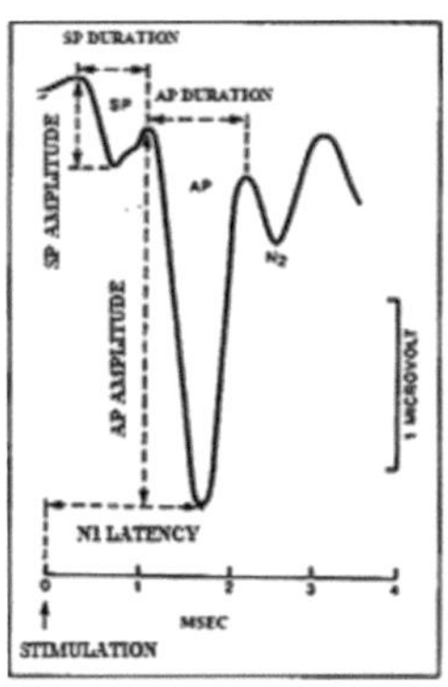

Figure 8. Global action potential.

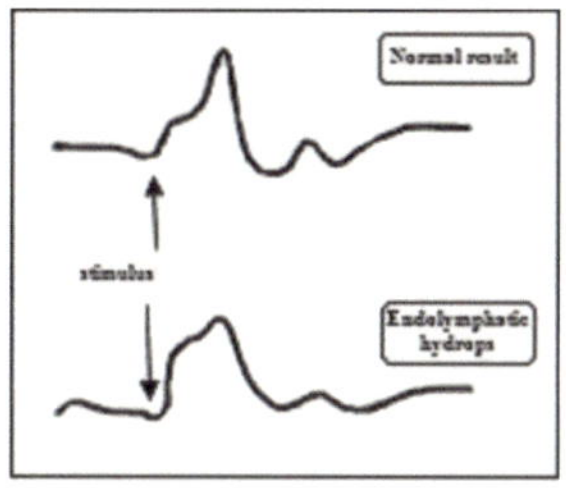

Figure 9. SP/AP amplitude ratio.

action potential. Magnitude of the AP compared with SP (SP/AP ratio) is increased in endolymphatic hydrops (>30%). The SP/AP amplitude ratio has 50–60% sensitivity in Ménière's disease diagnosis and 95% specificity in Refs. [11, 12] (**Figure 9**).

Recently, an area ratio (**Figure 10**) seems to be a more sensitive parameter for detecting endolymphatic hydrops [13]. An increase of more than 2 of SP/AP area together with the increase of SP/AP amplitude ratio increases sensitivity and specificity in Menière's disease diagnosis to 92 and 83.9%, respectively [14]. Some EP machines enabled automatically measurement of the area ratio.

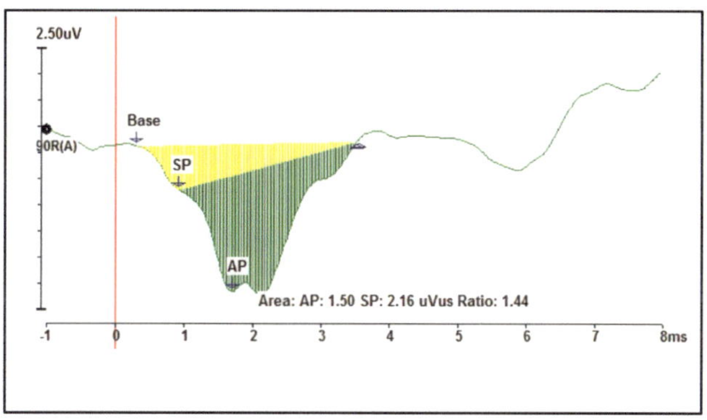

Figure 10. SP/AP area ratio (www.nervecenter.natus.com).

3. Vestibular evaluation

Vestibular investigations are also recommended in Menière's disease patients not only as a recommended battery test for positive diagnosis, but also in order to evaluate the degree of vestibular lesion which is present from the beginning of the Menière's disease.

Both vestibulo-ocular reflex (VOR) and vestibulospinal reflex (VSR) should be evaluated. Besides bed-side evaluation, objective vestibular tests are performed for a quantitative measure of these two vestibular reflexes useful in understanding the vestibular deficits as the disease proceeds.

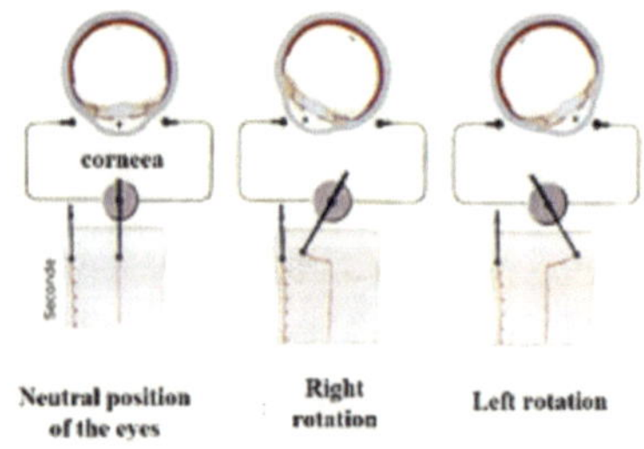

Figure 11. Nystagmus recording = variations of the corneo-retinian potential.

3.1. Vestibulo-ocular reflex

3.1.1. Electronystagmography (ENG)/videonystagmography (VNG)

Electro- or videonystagmography allows quantification of the nystagmus, as specific sign of vestibule-ocular reflex dysfunction. Nystagmus, as a conjugate movement of eyes with a slow and a fast phase provoked by vestibular asymmetry, reflects variations of the corneo-retinian potential during eyes movement (**Figure 11**). The slow phase is the effect of vestibular stimulation and its amplitude is proportional to the intensity of vestibular stimulation. The fast phase is central in origin and reflects only the reflex movement of the eyes to return to their normal position in the orbit. The fast phase direction gives the nystagmus direction.

The corneo-retinian potential can be measured by surface electrodes fixed around the eyes, horizontal and vertical or registered with infrared camera (**Figure 12**) in Refs. [15–17]. Conventionally, for horizontal electrodes, the upward fast phase is considered right beating nystagmus, while the downward fast phase is considered left beating nystagmus. For vertical electrodes, the upward fast phase is considered superior beating nystagmus, while the downward fast phase is considered inferior beating nystagmus.

Quantification of the nystagmus is based on several parameters:

- Direction of the nystagmus—linear, vertical, rotatory; right-, left-, superior- or inferior-beating nystagmus.
- Velocity of the slow phase, vestibular in origin (**Figure 12**).

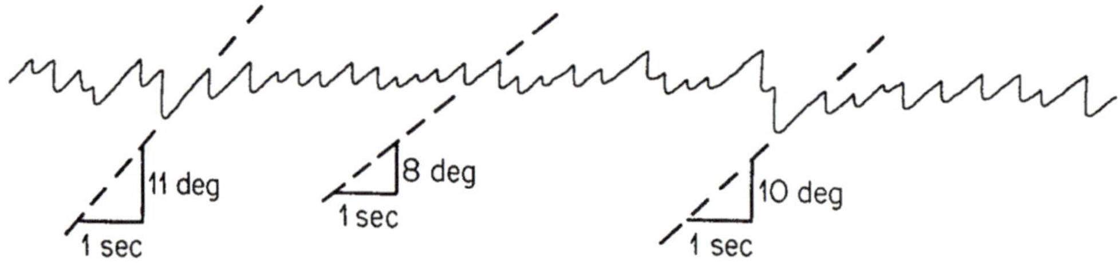

Figure 12. Calculation of nystagmus slow phase velocity.

Several tests are included in the electro-/videonystagmography (ENG/VNG): spontaneous nystagmus, positional, and positioning nystagmus, as well as provoked nystagmus (post or perrotatory nystagmus and caloric nystagmus). The provoked test is recommended only if patient is not in an acute vertigo phase.

Rotatory and caloric testing evaluates semicircular canal function in response to rotation or irrigation with warm and cold water/air of the external ear canal. Bithermal irrigation causes convective movement of endolymph in the ipsilateral horizontal semicircular canal, caloric test being the only available test that gives information regarding each horizontal semicircular canal. The movement of the endolymph provoked by variation of temperature and, secondary, endolymph density results in deflection of the cupula of the irrigated semicircular canal. Motion of the cupula leads to vestibular hair cell excitation or inhibition with consecutive change of the discharge rate in the superior vestibular nerve fibers. The difference between the excitatory and inhibitory discharge rates of the two superior vestibular nerves reaches the vestibular nuclei. From here compensatory eye movements are elicited (slow phase of nystagmus), followed by rapid corrective saccades (fast phase of nystagmus).

In Menière's disease patients, results in ENG/VNG differ depending on the phase (acute, subacute, or chronic) and the duration of the disease.

At the beginning of an acute phase, due to the minor ruptures in the Reissner's membrane and an increase of potassium concentration in the endolymph, the vestibular sensorial epithelium in the affected ear is stimulated and the spontaneous nystagmus beats toward the Menière's ear (**Figure 13**). Soon after, due to constantly increasing of the potassium concentration, the vestibular hair cells are intoxicated and their function decrease. In this stage, spontaneous nystagmus changes its direction toward the healthy ear.

In the next days after the acute spell of the Menière's disease results in rotatory and caloric test varies—either hypofunction in the affected ear (**Figure 14**), or symmetric functionality of the inner ears. The absence of a fixed vestibular lesion is the case in most of patients. In prolonged Menière's disease (long-term/chronic effect) usually patients' express caloric hypofunction of the affected ear (1/2—2/3 of patients) as VOR reflects the decreased input from the damaged

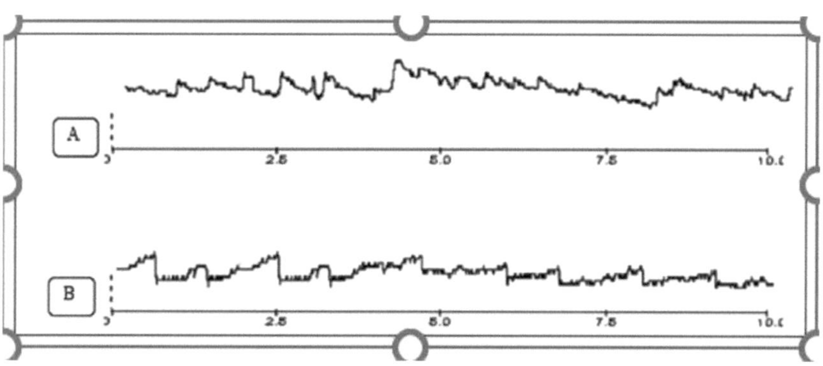

Figure 13. Spontaneous nystagmus: A—initial phase of the spell (towards the affected ear); B—end of the spell (towards the non-affected ear).

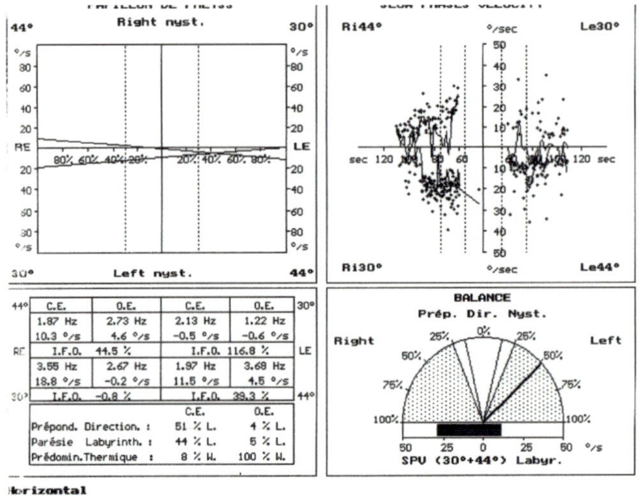

Figure 14. Left ear caloric hyporeflexia-hypofunction index > 30%.

ear. Caloric stimulation can be done sequential with warm and cold water, respectively, for each ear, or simultaneously. Bilateral cold water (30°C) irrigation shows rapidly the affected ear—the ear toward the nystagmus appears.

In rotatory chair test, results are usually normal. Directional preponderance is rarely seen, usually in long-duration Menière's disease, when vestibular lesion is stable at some extent (**Figure 15**). But immediately after an acute attack, VOR gain is increased in rotation toward the affected ear [18].

In between the acute spells, Menière's disease patients can experience positional vertigo, usually due to benign paroxysmal positional vertigo (BPPV). Disturbances in endolymph metabolism affect the function of the *stria vascularis* with secondary negative effects on the otolithic membrane. Still, BPPV is more frequently associated with vestibular migraine than Menière's disease.

3.1.2. Video head impulse test

The video head impulse test (HIT) evaluates as well semicircular canal function. Integrity of the VOR allows the tested subject to maintain sight fixed during high-acceleration high-velocity

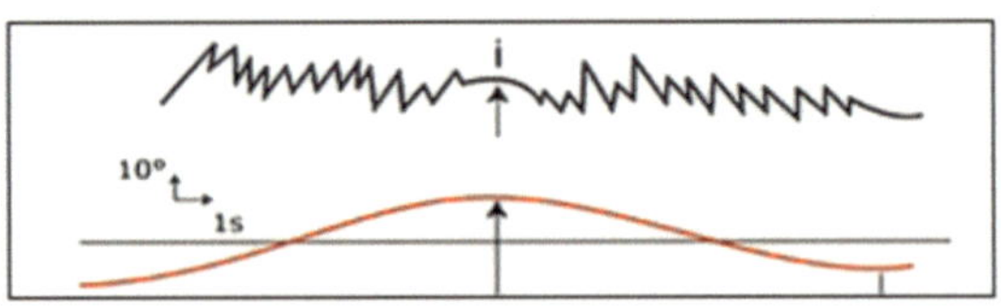

Figure 15. Symmetrical VOR response in rotatory test.

head rotations in space (gain values close to 1.0, as the ratio between eye and head velocity). Rotation is performed in each plane with an excitatory effect on each of the six semicircular canals.

A positive HIT stands for complete lesion of the fibers connected with the tested semicircular canal. In comparison with caloric testing, video HIT is abnormal in much more small numbers of Menière's disease patients, maybe because vestibular lesion is not complete.

3.2. Vestibulospinal reflex (VSR)

Equilibrium is a complex process, essential in human well-being and daily activities. It allows standing on different supports as well as walking and other movements without falling or disequilibrium.

Body and head position in space, related to gravity and environment landmarks (of verticality for example), is based on normal and correlated information's form sensorimotor, visual and vestibular systems. The most important, for sure until adult life, is the sensorimotor system—proprioceptors from feet and neck contribute mostly in equilibrium as we move in space.

As long as the child grows, visual information becomes more important in equilibrium, especially when visual surroundings are difficult.

A vestibular system develops in function in the first year of life and contributes progressively more to equilibrium. Its contribution increases in the case of a lesion in either of the other two systems [15–17]. Besides this, a severe unilateral vestibular deficit or bilateral vestibular lesion has a huge impact on equilibrium, at least for several weeks until a unilateral vestibular deficit is compensated by the other ear.

In Menière's disease, pathophysiology of the disease explains the fluctuating vestibular function of the affected ear. So, we do not have a stable deficit, at least not a complete one, or from the very beginning of the disease. For this reason, vestibular investigations have different results, from patient to patient, as we discussed in the ENG section.

3.2.1. Computerized dynamic posturography

Computerized dynamic posturography (CDP) contributes with specific parameters in monitoring patients with Menière's disease—for appropriate diagnostic and management. CDP is based on a force plate system capable of measuring the antero-posterior balance of the center of gravity of the tested subject and automatically compare this balance with normal values for patient's group of age.

Sensory organization test (SOT) is the most common test of CDP. It allows a selective use of each of the three systems involved in equilibrium during six different conditions of testing (**Figure 16**) in [19] and thus a global and selective evaluation of equilibrium, based on the system used for maintaining the standing position during testing in [20].

As long as projection of the center of gravity (COG) during testing is inside the base support area and no external support is used for stabilize, patient is able to maintain his/her equilibrium and normal result will be displayed at the end of the test (**Figure 17**). When patient

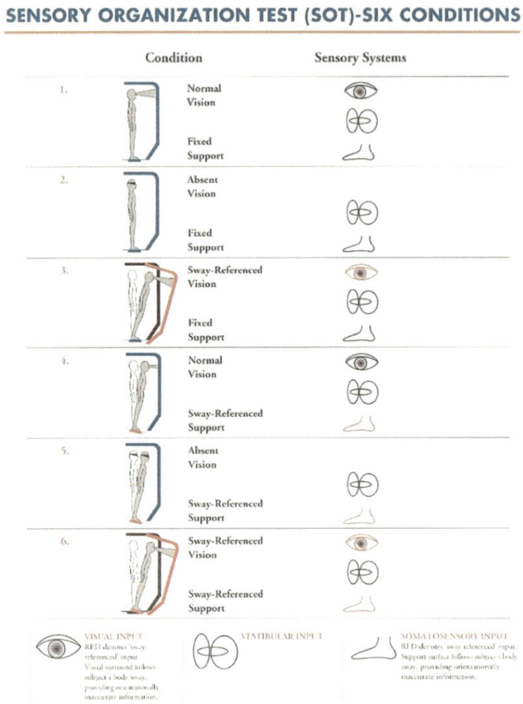

Figure 16. CDP/SOT testing conditions (www.nervecenter.natus.com).

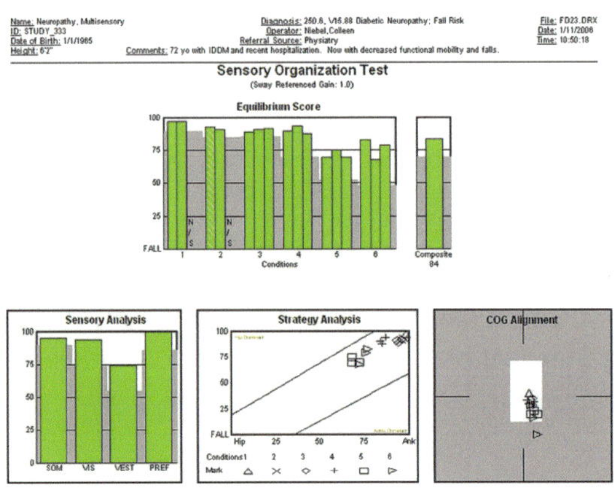

Figure 17. CDP—normal result.

cannot voluntary control its balance within the parameters described, he will obtain a pathological score of equilibrium, displayed at glance with colors convention and also with numeric values (**Figure 18**).

In Menière's disease patients, CDP usually display normal results, since in between the spells patient has no equilibrium problems and the acute vestibular deficit of the affected ear was

http://dx.doi.org/10.5772/66382

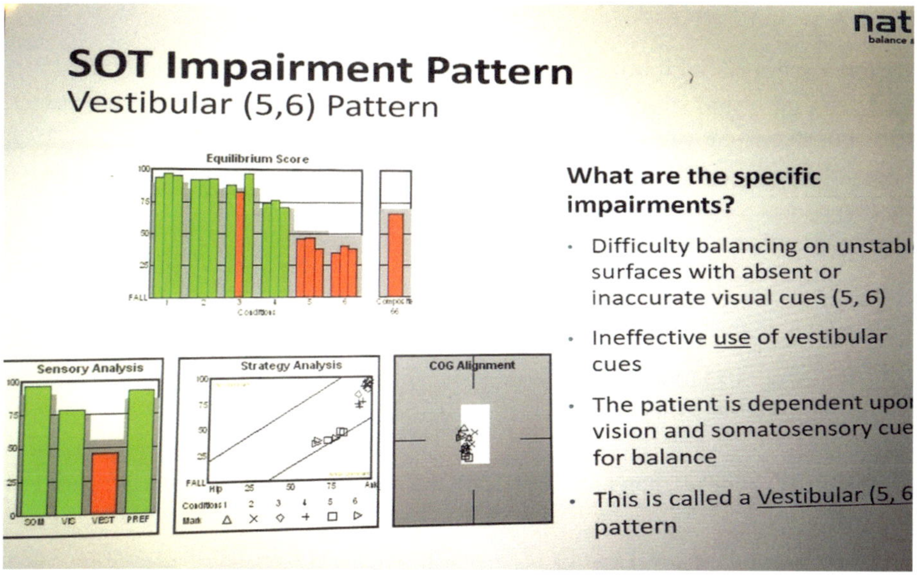

Figure 18. CDP—pathological result: vestibular deficit.

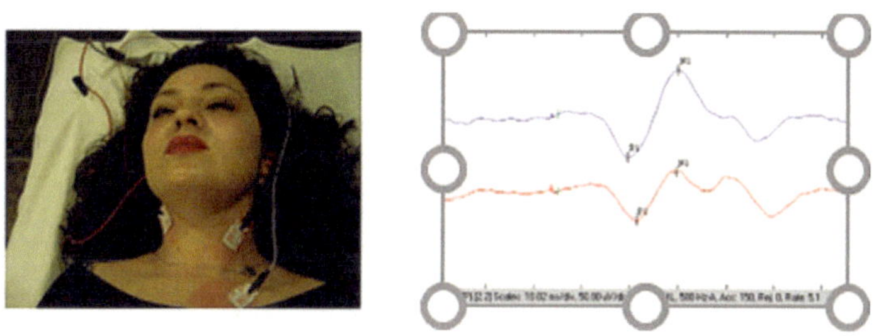

Figure 19. Montage and cVEMP biphasic potential.

compensated already. Immediately after the acute phase, vestibular scores can be abnormal, mainly in vestibular condition.

3.2.2. Vestibular evoked miogenic potentials

Vestibular evoked miogenic potentials (VEMPs) area relatively new objective test designed to measure otolithic function in [21]. In response to loud sound stimulation (95–97dB nHL), saccular vestibular sensorial epithelium generates activity in the inferior vestibular nerve and further in the vestibulospinal and vestibule-ocular pathway.

Action potential transmitted through the vestibulospinal pathway generates muscular responses in the effectors of the vestibulospinal (cervical muscles—cervical vestibular evoked myogenic potential: cVEMP) or vestibule-ocular reflex (extraocular muscles—ocular vestibular evoked myogenic potential: oVEMP).

3.2.2.1. Cervical VEMP

cVEMP represents an inhibitory biphasic response in the ipsilateral sternocleidomastoid muscle after loud sound stimulation of the sacculae, which can be recorded by surface electrodes. A positive-negative P13-N23 potential is recorded with normal latencies of 13 and 23 ms, respectively (**Figure 19**). The greatest sensitivity of sacculocolic reflex is for 200–1000 Hz stimuli in Refs. [22, 23], a frequency range highly correlated with saccular function and resonance properties as well (which are correlated with saccular size).

Late N34-P44 potentials are not saccular in origins. The amplitude of the response varies with contraction level of the muscle (**Figure 20**).

A clinical value of cVEMP is based on comparison of cVEMP amplitude in response to each saccular stimulation. For this reason, contraction level should be measure as well and rectified traces are evaluated. A difference of more than 30% between cVEMP amplitudes is considered abnormal, in result either to saccular hypofunction or hyperfunction depending on the pathology.

In Menière's disease, endolymphatic hydrops involves the sacculae from the very initial stages of the disease with secondary variations in sacculae's mechanical properties. Since cervical VEMP depends on the physical characteristics of the sacculae, cVEMP is included in the vestibular battery test for Menière's disease diagnosis. In more than 50% of Menière's disease patients, click-evoked cVEMP is abnormal or absent in Refs. [24, 25].

It also has been studied frequency tuning of cVEMP in endolymphatic hydrops and it appears that VEMP is recorded at higher frequencies and across broader frequency ranges than in normal inner ears due to changes in saccular resonance characteristics [26].

These two changes (blunting and frequency shift of cVEMP) are greater as the Menière's disease has a longer evolution and greater severity in [27]. Additionally, over 20% of Menière's disease patients have abnormal cVEMP results in the non-affected ear in Ref. [28], recommending VEMP as a predictor test for bilateral Menière's disease.

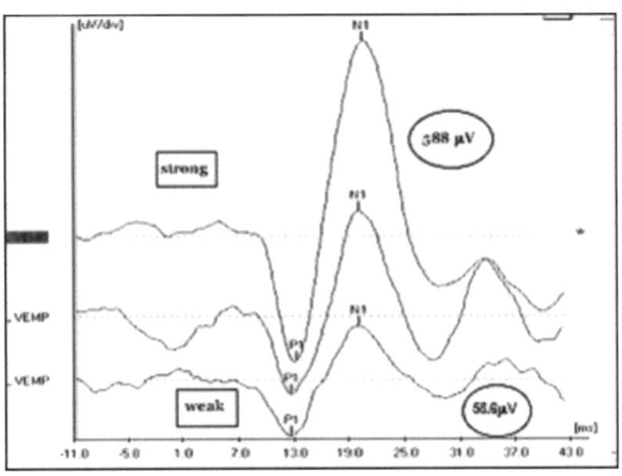

Figure 20. Amplitude variation in relation with muscle contraction.

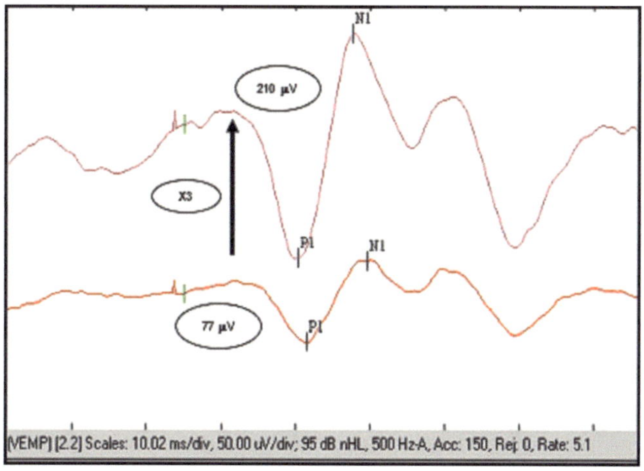

Figure 21. VEMP amplitude variation in positive glycerol test.

Another study revealed a correlation between cVEMP threshold variations in between affected and nonaffected ear and the severity of Menière's disease in Ref. [29].

In a small series of Menière's disease patients, VEMP increased in amplitude, even three times at the end of positive glycerol test (**Figure 21**) as an argument of presence of the endolymphatic hydrops in the sacculae in Ref. [30].

3.2.2.2. Ocular VEMP

Ocular VEMP (oVEMP) is a newer variant of VEMP which measures saccular function in response to very loud sound stimulation (about 120–130 dB SPL) or utricular function in response to vibrations applied to the cochlea. Electrodes placed below the orbit record excitatory response in the contralateral inferior oblique muscle when in a flexed state by looking upward in Ref. [31].

The first negative (excitatory) component of the oVEMP at a latency of about 10 ms is called n10. This n10 component most likely indicates the myogenic potentials of inferior oblique muscle.

Additionally, in patients with early Menière's disease tested at attack, the contralateral oVEMP n10 is enhanced compared to measures in the same patients at quiescence. We speculate that this enhancement by Menière's disease attack could be due to mechanical changes in the labyrinth that enhance the sensitive response of utricular receptors to bone conduction vibrator stimulation. It seems that alterations in frequency tuning discussed in cVEMP are also present in sound-evoked oVEMP in Menière's disease patients in Ref. [32].

Author details

Madalina Gabriela Georgescu

Address all correspondence to: madalina.georgescu@gecad.com

"Carol Davila" University of Medicine and Pharmacy, Bucharest, Romania

References

[1] Hulshof JH, Baarsma EA. Vestibular investigations in Menière's disease. Acta Otolaryngol 1981;92:75-81.

[2] Bronstein AM. Oxford Textbook of Vertigo and Imbalance. UK: Oxford University Press; 2013, pp. 243-244.

[3] Dix MR, Hallpike CS, Hood JD. Observations upon the loudness recruitment phenomenon, with special reference to the differential diagnosis of disorders of the internal ear and eight nerve. Proc R Soc Med 1948;41(8):516-526.

[4] Dix MR, Hallpike CS. The otoneurological diagnosis of tumours of the VIII nerve. Proc R Soc Med 1958;51(11):889-896.

[5] Hood DJ. Loudness balance procedures for the measurement of recruitment. Audiology 1977;16(3):215-228.

[6] Pascu A. Audiometry (Romanian language). Romania: "Carol Davila" University ed.; 2000, 205 p.

[7] Pascu A. ABR in retrocochlear lesion diagnosis [PhD thesis] (Romanian language). Bucharest: University of Medicine and Pharmacy; 1995.

[8] American Speech-Language-Hearing Association (ASHA). The Short Latency Auditory Evoked Potentials. Rockville Pike, MD: ASHA; 1987.

[9] Ruth RA, Lambert PR, Ferraro JA. Electrocochleography: methods and clinical applications. Am J Otol 1988;9(Suppl):1-11.

[10] Abbas PJ, Brown CJ. Electrocochleography, In: Katz J, Burkard RF, Medwetsky L, (eds.), Handbook of Clinical Audiology. 6th ed. Philadelphia, OA: Lippincott, Williams & Wilkins; 2009, pp. 265-292.

[11] Sass K. Sensitivity and specificity of transtympanic electrocochleography in Meniere's disease. Acta Otolaryngol 1998;118(2):150-156.

[12] Chung WH, Cho DY, Choi JY, Hong SH. Clinical usefulness of extratympanic electrocochleography in the diagnosis of Meniere's disease. Otol Neurotol 2004;25(2):144-149.

[13] Devaiah AK, Dawson KL, Ferraro JA, Ator GA. Utility of area curve ratio electrocochleography in early Meniere's disease. Arch Otolaryngol Head Neck Surg 2003;129(5):547-551.

[14] Al-Momani M, Ferraro J, Ator G, Gajewski B. Improved sensitivity of ECochG in the diagnosis of Menière's disease. Int J Audiol 2009;48:811-819.

[15] Fluur E, Mellström A. Dynamic body stabilization: EquiTest system in patients with bilateral vestibular caloric areflexia. In: Woollacott M, Horak F, (eds.), Posture and Gait: Control Mechanisms vol. I, Eugene, OR: Eugene University of Oregon Books, ; 1992, pp. 292-295.

[16] Georgescu M. Evaluation of the dizzy patient (Romanian language). Bucharest: Mayko ed.; 2005, 351 p.

[17] Goebel JA, Paige GD. Dynamic posturography and caloric test results in patients with and without vertigo. Otolaryngol Head Neck Surg 1989;100:553-558.

[18] Alpert JN, Coats AC, Perusquia E. Saccadic nystagmus in cortical cerebellar atrophy. Neurology 1975;25:276-280.

[19] WWW–www.nervecenter.natus.com

[20] Brodal A. Anatomical studies of cerebellar fiber connections with special reference to problems of functional localization. In Schade JP, (ed.), The Cerebellum, vol 25, Progress in Brain Research. Amsterdam: Elsevier Publishing Co; 1967.

[21] Halmagyi GM, Colebatch JG, Curthoys IS. New tests of vestibular function. Baillieres Clin Neurol 1994;3:485-500.

[22] Todd NP, Cody FW, Banks JR. A saccular origin of frequency tuning in myogenic vestibular evoked potentials? Implications for human responses to loud sounds. Hear Res 2000;141(102):180-188.

[23] Wegampola MS, Colebatch JG. Characteristics of tone burst-evoked myogenic potentials in the sternocleidomastoid muscles. Otol Neurotol 2001;22(6):796-802.

[24] de Waele C, Huy PT, Diard JP, Freyss G, Vidal PP. Saccular dusfunction in Meniere's disease. Am J Otol 1999;20(2):223-232.

[25] Murofushi T, Shimizu K, Takegoshi H, Cheng PW. Diagnostic value of prolonged latencies in the vestibular myogenic potential. Arch Otolaryngol Head Neck Surg 2001;127(9):1069-1072.

[26] Rauch SD, Zhou G, Kujawa SG, Guinan JJ, Herrmann BS. Vestibular evoked myogenic potentials show altered tuning in patients with Meniere's disease. Otol Neurotol 2004;25(3):333-338.

[27] Timmer FC, Zhou G, Guinan JJ, Kujawa SG, Herrmann BS, Rauch SD. Vestibular evoked myogenic potential (VEMP) in patients with Meniere's disease with drop attacks. Laryngoscope 2006;116(5):776-779.

[28] Lin MY, Timmer FC, Oriel BS, et al. Vestibular evoked myogenic potentials (VEMP) can detect asymptomatic saccular hydrops. Laryngoscope 2006;116(6):987-992.

[29] Young YH, Huang TW, Cheng PW. Assessing the stage of Meniere's disease using vestibular evoked myogenic potentials. Arch Otolaryngol Head Neck Surg 2003;129(8):815-818.

[30] Georgescu M, Cernea M. Clinical value of VEMP in Meniere's disease diagnosis (Romanian language). ORL.ro 2014;6(23):14-26.

[31] Rosengren SM, Todd NM, Colebatch JG. Vestibularevoked extraocular potentials produced by stimulation with bone-conducted sound. Clin Neurophysiol 2005;116(8):1938-1948.

[32] Winters SM, Berg IT, Grolman W, Klis SF. Ocular vestibular evoked myogenic potentials: Frequency tuning to airconducted acoustic stimuli in healthy subjects and Meniere's disease. Audiol Neurotol 2012;17(1):12-19.

Chapter 9

Testing of the Semicircular Canal Function in Vertigo and Dizziness

Holger A. Rambold

Additional information is available at the end of the chapter

http://dx.doi.org/10.5772/66688

Abstract

Testing the function of the semicircular canals (SCC) in vertigo and dizziness is an important step towards a diagnosis. There are different vestibular tests available: rotatory testing, bithermal caloric irrigation (CI) and the video-head-impulse test (vHIT). This chapter describes the basic methods, the current knowledge and economic aspects focused on the vHIT and CI. After a general section, common vertigo diseases are discussed with respect to the functional tests. From this chapter, it is clear that not only one method has to be applied to test vestibular function but a battery including the CI and the vHIT in three dimensions.

Keywords: video-head-impulse test, bithermal caloric irrigation, vestibular tests, vertigo, dizziness, vestibular disease

1. Introduction

One major step in diagnosing dizziness and vestibular disease, in addition to a detailed clinical history and neurologic, neuro-ophthalmologic and neuro-otologic examination, is to test the sensors of the labyrinth quantitatively. There are two sets of sensors: the linear/gravity sensors (otoliths, sacculus and utriculus) and the rotational sensors (semicircular canals; SSCs). Both sensor types are important to keep balance and help to orient oneself in space. To test the sensors, different specific tests are available and it is often unclear what methods should be used. This chapter summarizes current knowledge of the testing opportunities and techniques in respect to vestibular function of the SCCs and to different disease. First the different techniques, second the lesion patterns in different vertigo/dizziness disease and third economic aspects are described.

INTECH
open science | open minds

© 2017 The Author(s). Licensee InTech. This chapter is distributed under the terms of the Creative Commons Attribution License (http://creativecommons.org/licenses/by/3.0), which permits unrestricted use, distribution, and reproduction in any medium, provided the original work is properly cited. (cc) BY

2. Testing of the SCCs

2.1. Anatomical and physiological basics

The SCCs are part of the three-neuron reflex that stabilizes the eyes in space during rotatory self motion, the vestibulo-ocular reflex (VOR). The VOR is quantified as a gain, the ratio of eye-to-head velocity. During normal functioning, the VOR gain is one; eye and head move in opposite direction but with equal velocity [1]. The reflex starts at the sensors, the three SCCs, which are located on each side of the head in the temporal bone. While the horizontal SCCs (HC) are found in a slightly upward tilted horizontal plane (30°), the vertical SCCs are orthogonal to the HC. The SCCs are located in the sagittal plane, which is rotated 45° to either the right or the left. Accordingly, there are two anterior (AC) and two posterior SCCs (PC) found. The main stimulus for the SCCs is the rotational acceleration around an axis orthogonal to the canals plane.

The SCCs are stimulated by the endolymphatic flow relative to the crista ampullaris which is caused by the inertia during rotational stimuli [1]. This flow causes the crista ampullaris to be deflected. Endolymphatic flow in the HC in direction to the ampulla (ampullopetal) causes excitation and away from the ampulla (ampullofugal) inhibition. It is important to mention that in case of the vertical SCCs this direction is inversed.

Neuronal signals originating in the crista ampullaris are transferred to the vestibular nuclei by the vestibular nerve. This nerve has a steady-state neuronal firing rate of about 100 spike/s at rest [1]. Excitation of the SCCs can increase the spike rate up to about 400 spikes/s, inhibition of the SCCs decreases the spike rate, but no less than zero spikes/s [2].

The vestibular nerve has two divisions: the superior receives afferents from the utriculus, the horizontal and anterior SCC, the inferior division from the sacculus and the posterior semi-circular canals. Some details are still discussed controversial, for example, if the sacculus projection to the superior vestibular nerve division is of clinical relevance [1].

2.2. Different methods

2.2.1. Rotatory tests

Testing the SCCs could be obtained by passive rotational stimuli which both labyrinths together. This kind of test has been applied for years, but the sensitivity to identify unilateral vestibular failure is low. The test depends on the velocity profile, the disease itself, the stage of the disease, the cooperation and alertness of the patients [1, 3–8]. By analysing the postrotatory response to step stimuli not only side differences but additionally the central processing of the VOR, including the 'velocity storage', could be quantified [9]. The 'velocity storage' is known as the indirect pathway, which acts parallel to the direct VOR pathway [10] and is realized by a commissural inhibitory network [11–14] under cerebellar control of the uvula and nodulus [15]. One function of the 'velocity storage' is to increase the cupula time constant to improve the ability to transduce the low-frequency components of the VOR [16]. Other functions of the 'velocity storage' are to reorient the eye velocity in direction of the gravitoinertial acceleration and to differentiate linear acceleration from gravity [9]. Remember, these rotational tests have special advantages for certain disease, but examine only the two horizontal SCCs of the right and the left inner ear together. Furthermore, the rotational chairs are currently to slow and the available eye movement-recording systems are very restricted in spatial and temporal resolution, to stimulate just one SCC.

2.2.2. *Bithermal caloric test (CI)*

A common test to test the horizontal SCCs *unilaterally* is the bithermal caloric irrigation (CI). For describing the mechanism of the caloric test, Róbert Bárány received the Nobel Prize in Medicine in 1916. This test uses a very low-frequency range, is not physiological, but important in a vestibular test battery. Remember, this test was the standard test to diagnose vestibular hypofunction before modern commercial methods became available around 2010.

The response of the horizontal SCCs to thermal irrigation depends on the amount of thermal energy which reaches the inner ear to elicit the VOR. Depending on the anatomy or disease, the thermal conductance through the middle and inner ear could be different.

There are two mechanisms discussed to elicit the caloric response. The major response is caused by temperature-induced endolymphatic flow, the other by a direct thermal stimulation of the vestibular nerve. The latter was identified in microgravity during space flight [17, 18].

The test protocol is standardized, but normative values should be measured in each laboratory separately. Caloric bithermal testing is performed in the supine position with the head flexed 30° upward to orient the horizontal SCCs vertically [19]. Irrigation of the external auditory duct of each ear is performed with water at a temperature of 30 or 44°C for 1 min. In between the irrigations, there is an interval of at least 5 min. To obtain a side difference between the right and left ear, the unilateral weakness is calculated using the best responses of the slow-phase velocities with the Jongkees formula: $UW = ((RW + RC) - (LW + LC))/(RW + LW + RC + LC) \times 100$ (R: right; L: left ear ; water at 44°C (warm, W) and 30°C (cold, C)) [19]. In our laboratory, a value of 25% or higher is pathological. To measure directional asymmetry, the directional preponderance (DP) is quantified ($DP = ((RW - LW) - (RC - LC))/(RW + LW + RC + LC) \times 100$) [19]. Normal values in our laboratory are up to 30% (absolute values).

It is known from various studies that the sensitivity and specificity are higher in bithermal compared to monothermal irrigations [20, 21]. In our laboratory, we have a sensitivity of 80%, a specificity of 81% and a false-negative rate of 21% for bithermal versus monothermal CI. Monothermal CI could not be applied efficiently if the maximal caloric slow-phase velocities are below 11°/s or if nystagmus is present [22]. The false-negative rate, which ranges in the literature from 10 to 30%, as in our study, precludes the routine use [22, 23].

Another question, which is also discussed, is whether air or water should be used for optimal CI. One major problem was the high test-retest variability of air irrigation [24]. The problem is the amount of thermal energy to be transferred through the middle to the inner ear to elicit the VOR. Hence, higher and lower temperatures compared to water irrigation can be used in air irrigation in order to achieve comparable results [25]. Other and our laboratory prefer still water irrigation for the obvious reasons [26].

2.2.3. Video-head-impulse test (vHIT)

In 1988, M. Halmagyi published the first report of a clinical bedside test to evaluate the horizontal SCCs. This test is known as the 'Halmagyi-test', the 'Halmagyi-Curthoys test' or the 'head-impulse test.' In this test, high-acceleration, small-amplitude head pulses around an earth-vertical axis are applied while the patient is fixating a stationary target. If the eye no longer compensates the head movement, a correcting saccade is observed and the test is rated pathologic. This bedside test (bHIT) for the HC does not identify all unilateral vestibular failures. It has a moderate sensitivity (35–45%) and a high specificity (90%) [27, 28]. To achieve better sensitivity and specificity than the bHIT, the HIT measured with a video system (vHIT) was developed [29–31]. The increase in sensitivity and specificity is mainly attributed to the fact that correcting saccades are clearly identified and the VOR gain can be measured. The vHIT has been shown to be comparable to those HIT measurements with the complicated and time-consuming scleral-search-coil technique [32]. There are meanwhile several companies which sell measuring devices based on video oculography (e.g. GN-Otometrics®, EyeSee-Cam®, Synapsis®, Firefly MV® and Vorteque®).

In contrast to the bHIT, the examiner stands behind the patient during the vHIT, while the patient fixates a point in 1-m distance at the wall. Eye movements are recorded in most systems by a small video camera mounted in goggles worn by the patient during the test. This modern vestibular test examines not only the HC but also the AC and the PC to identify unilateral or bilateral vestibular (BV) hypofunction of individuals SCCs [33]. The direction of the head movements defines the SCC stimulated. Rotating the head around an earth vertical axis to the right or left tests the right or left HC, rotating around an earth horizontal axis (forward and backward) while the head is constantly turned by 45° to the right or left around an earth vertical axis, activates either the right AC or left PC (RALP) or the left AC or right PC (LARP).

It is critically important to reach high enough head acceleration and velocities values to obtain valid examinations. Velocities of 200–250°/s for the horizontal and 150°/s for the vertical vHIT are recommended. To reach such values is sometimes a problem in older patients with high muscle tone in the neck. Patients with neck problems, especially degenerative disease of the cervical spine, should not be tested in order to avoid injuring the patient [31].

In case of a pathological test, the gain is decreased and refixating saccades (RFSs) are observed [33, 34]. For each different company selling vHIT measuring devices, there are different normative values for the gains. The cut-off values are about 0.8 for horizontal and 0.6 for vertical vHIT. These values might decrease with an increasing age in some but not all studies and depending on the type of measuring device used [35–40]. RFS might occur during the head impulse or after the end of the head impulse and are referred to as covert and overt RFS [29]. RFSs are much more reliable than the VOR gain values in between different testers [41]. One problem is RFS, which increase in higher age without a VOR gain decrease and could clinically mimic a pathological vHIT [35]. To diagnose a vestibular hypofunction with a vHIT a low VOR gain, compensatory RFS and an optimally performance of the head impulses are necessary.

2.2.4. Differences between CI and vHIT

Both tests measure unilateral HC but in different ways. Therefore, it is clear that the overall sensitivity and specificity for a unilateral failure are different. Measuring such parameters needs a golden standard, which is hard to define as both tests are important on their own.

The vHIT compared to the CI has an overall sensitivity of 41% and a specificity of 92% which is very similar to data of the bHIT in comparison to the CI (sensitivity of 35%; specificity of 95–100% [27, 28]). It is known that the probability of a pathologic bHIT increases with UW and that a UW of 42.5% ensures a pathological bHIT [31, 42]. Our data support this finding also for the vHIT. A unilateral weakness of 57% was observed in the pathological vHIT and 42% in the normal vHIT group. The vHIT is also affected by the disease stage (acute versus non-acute). The frequency of vHIT increases with increasing UW for all patients but more for the acute subgroup compared to the non-acute subgroup [31].

Why the two tests dissociate is controversially discussed. The vHIT and CI might test the VOR at different temporal frequencies, the HIT tests high frequencies up to 5 Hz [43] and the CI tests the lower frequency range at about 0.003 Hz. Stimulation of control subjects on a rotatory chair around an earth vertical axis at 0.003 Hz does not cause the slow-phase velocities obtained by CI (personal communication D. Straumann). One reason for this difference might be attributed to the fact that CI also stimulates the nerve directly [44]. There is some evidence from animal experiments that different vestibular nerve fibres might be important. Higher gains at low frequency are found in regular vestibular afferent fibres and higher gains at higher frequencies in irregular fibres [45]. The contribution of the different fibres to vestibular function and the vHIT and CI remains unclear at the moment [46].

There is another explanation discussed, which could explain different findings. During endolymphatic hydrops, the diameter of the semicircular duct expands, which might lead to an endolymphatic circulation in the duct itself. This results in a lowered or absent caloric response, but an unremarkable vHIT [47].

2.3. Specific disease

2.3.1. Vestibular neuritis (VN)

In vestibular neuritis (VN), mostly an ipsilesional UW and a pathological horizontal vHIT is found. There are, however, sometimes differences in the results of a pathological UW and horizontal vHIT [31, 48–50]. In a series including acute, not acute and follow-up VN patients, we found 47% with a pathological horizontal vHIT and UW (>25%), 25% with a pathological UW only and 8% with an isolated pathological vHIT. In an earlier case series using the scleral-search-coil technique and defining the pathological HIT by the VOR-gain only, all patients with VN had a pathological HIT. In the acute, but not in the late stage, there was also an UW (100 vs. 64%) [51]. The pathological vHIT and UW are not correlated with the clinical picture and symptoms [31, 49]. The time course of recovery of vHIT and UW and was also not correlated in a retrospective study after the onset of VN [50]. In a pathological vHIT covert or overt RFSs are observed. To link the different correcting saccade patterns to clinical outcome has failed so far [50, 52].

The advantage of the three-dimensional (3-D) vHIT is additionally to test the AC and PC. One can therefore differentiate the lesion based on the affected SCCs in an inferior (PC), superior (HC and AC) or combined VN. In studies, the lesion pattern was shown to be in the superior in 90–48%, inferior in 1–18% and combined inferior and superior vestibular nerve divisions in 34% of the patients [53–56]. The lesion pattern affects the outcome. It was shown that the time to recovery increased from inferior over superior to combined VN [54].

UW without a vHIT is often found in patients of higher age (mean age 64 years) and without a history of Meniere disease (MD) as a first time acute vestibular syndrome. The disease is undefined and might be caused by an endolymphatic hydrops or an incomplete VN. Patients with such a lesion pattern are hospitalized for less time than patients with an additional pathological horizontal vHIT [56].

2.3.2. Meniere disease (MD)

In general, during an attack, there is a decreased UW (64–67%) on the affected side [57, 58], which is caused by the endolymphatic hydrops by an expanse of the endolymph volume, which led to local circulation of the thermal-induced endolymphatic flow [47]. The results of the vHIT are contradictory. The horizontal VOR gain of the affected ear might be mostly slightly reduced [57], or in some cases be increased [59]. During the hydrops, there might be an increase in VOR gain in the vHIT (14%), it might be either normal (67%) or decreased (19%) in the healthy ear [57]. The VOR gains for the AC and PC did not differ between the sides during the attacks [57]. In between the attacks, the vHIT was normal in 33%, pathologic of at least one SCC on the affected side in 33% and pathologic in one SCC on the affected and unaffected side in 31%. The distribution of abnormal findings was dependent on the disease duration and hearing loss [60]. In summary, the findings of CI and vHIT are heterogeneous.

2.3.3. Vestibular migraine (VM)

Vestibular migraine (VM) is a disease which could be confused with MD. To make it even more complicated, there is high co-morbidity of the two diseases and it is sometimes hard to come up with a diagnosis [61]. Vestibular and oculomotor tests could be in between the VM attacks pathological [20, 62, 63] but vestibular dysfunction is not a prognostic factor for migraine patients [64].

To dissociate both diseases based on the CI and vHIT in early or late stage is not possible. An UW and vHIT pathology is more often found in MD (67 and 37%) compared to VM (22 and 9%) [58]. In general, the caloric peak slow-phase velocity values tend to be elevated in VM patients compared to MD [65, 66]. Remember, there is also a portion of common migraine patients which have a UW in between the attacks (16%) [67].

2.3.4. Vestibular schwannoma (VS)

The vestibular schwannoma (VS) can be divided in the intracochlear (50%), the vestibular type (19%) and more diffuse forms (31%). Deafness was the most common symptom and caloric tests were abnormal in 78% of cases. In the vestibular type, hearing was significant, but vestibular function was more altered [68]. It was shown that even very small and localized VS heavily compromise labyrinthine functions [68, 69]. VS initially show a pathological UW and a normal vHIT. However, with increasing size the vHIT might become pathological [69–71]. It is controversially discussed if UW is a predictor for tumour size [70, 72] or not [73]. It was shown that the VOR gain of vHIT is not correlated with the tumour size [70] but rated together with the CI there was a correlation. [71].

The 3-D vHIT might indicate some more information in conjunction with vestibular-evoked potentials (VEMPs). In a study on 50 patients, 58% of patients had test abnormalities which were referable to both superior and inferior vestibular nerve divisions. Selective inferior nerve dysfunction was identified in 10% and superior in 13%, indicating that lesions of the superior and inferior vestibular nerve evolved in parallel. The sensitivity of the test battery increased with tumour size and all patients with medium to large schwannoma had at least two abnormal vestibular test results [74]. From this finding, it might be clinically useful to use a more extended test battery and not a single test.

2.3.5. Sudden sensorineural hearing loss (SSNHL)

In contrast to the VN, which mostly affects the HC and AC, the lesion pattern in hearing loss is different. In a study on acute sensorineural hearing loss, 14% had a complete vestibular loss defined as involvement of all three SCCs, 31% a partial vestibular loss defined as involvement of one or two SCCs and 55% no measurable SCC loss. In the group with a partial lesion, all patients had the PC affected [75]. In another study on acute unilateral hearing loss *with* vestibular symptoms, there is an impairment of the PC in 74%, of the HC in 41% and of the AC in 30% [76]. Comparable data for CI were in both studies not available.

2.3.6. Bilateral vestibular (BV) failure

Recently, a caloric hypofunction of both ears (sum of all four best slow-phase velocity responses has to be less than 20°/s with bithermal CI) and deficits in rotatory tests were recommended to diagnose a BV [77]. With the current vHIT, which often clearly diagnoses a BV [78], things get more complicated. A consensus was reached on a pathological vHIT on both sides in addition to a caloric hypofunction to diagnose a BV and will be published in the newest form from the Barany Society soon (personal communication Prof. Dr. M. Strupp). These criteria are suboptimal; the vestibular organ could be hypo-responsive only to certain head frequency ranges, which make a rotatory testing necessary. Positive bilateral vHIT does not always correlate with caloric or rotatory chair test results in BV. This indicates that a spectrum of vestibulopathies exists according to the stimulation frequency of the deficit [79].

The results of the 3D-vHIT are very scattered with respect to SCC pathology [80]. In one current publication, the 3-D vHIT was characterized in a group including different aetiologies of BV.

The PC was most affected (89%), less the HC (85%) and least the AC (39%). Preserved AC function was associated with aminoglycoside toxicity, MD and BVL of unknown origin. No such sparing of specific SCCs was found for inner ear infections, cerebellar ataxia with neuropathy and bilateral vestibular areflexia syndrome (CANVAS) and sensorineural hearing loss [81]. CANVAS is a late-onset ataxia with a neuropathy and a BV [82].

2.3.7. Inferior cerebellar stroke

Stroke with an acute vestibular syndrome is found in about 16% of inferior cerebellar stroke. The main question is how to dissociate stroke from a peripheral vestibular lesion, which accounts for about 25% [83]. This is very important for stroke treatment as there is only a short time frame (4.5 h after symptom onset in Germany) to apply revascularization therapy with the systemic intravenous thrombolysis.

To differentiate the peripheral disease from stroke, the horizontal vHIT is used, together with central signs, for example, the gaze evoked nystagmus and the tonic skew deviation, a vertical divergence of the eyes. This test battery is also known as the HINTS test. In general, the vHIT is normal in stroke. There are some rare exceptions with lesions of the brainstem (e.g. vestibular nuclei) or cerebellum, mostly in the territory of the anterior inferior cerebellar artery (AICA). It is important that the auditory artery is a branch of the AICA which supplies the labyrinth and cochlea. For further discussion on this topic, I recommend the current literature [83–86].

3. Economic aspects

The CI nor the vHIT could replace each other. On the average, the time needed to perform a horizontal vHIT is 6 ± 1 min (mean ± standard deviation), 3-D vHIT 10 ± 2 min and a caloric irrigation 22 ± 2 min. The examination and documentation of the results by the clinician including removing error traces and setting markers right were estimated at 5–10 min for each test. Rotatory tests, which are more time consuming (10–20 min), might be important in only limited number of disease, for example, BV or central vestibular disease, which is not reviewed in detail here.

In certain disease and depending on the question, not all tests have to be applied, to save time. The saved time could be used to diagnose additional patients. From an economic point of view, just to identify a unilateral vestibular failure and with the mixture of diagnosis in a specialized vertigo/dizziness clinic, I recommend using the vHIT-first approach. In case of an unremarkable vHIT, you additionally should use the CI. There is one exception, if you clinically suspect an MD, you should use the CI first (for details see [20]). From these data, I suggest a disease-dependent approach to save diagnostic time and decrease stress of the patient.

4. Summary

From the reviewed data presented here, it is recommended to use a vestibular-testing battery depending on the question asked. The bithermal CI does not replace the vHIT and vice versa, both techniques are needed. In future, the more detailed vestibular test profiles will help to diagnose disease with a higher sensitivity and specificity, to predict outcome and to identify new disease with new therapeutic options.

Author details

Holger A. Rambold

Address all correspondence to: h.rambold@krk-aoe.de

Department of Neurology, County Hospitals of Altötting and Burghausen, Altötting, Germany

Department of Neurology, University of Regensburg, Regensburg, Germany

References

[1] Baloh RW, Honrubia V, Kerber KA. Baloh and Honrubias Clinical Neurophysiology of the Vestibular System. Oxford, New York, NY: Oxford University Press; 2011.

[2] Goldberg JM, Fernandez C. Physiology of peripheral neurons innervating semicircular canals of the squirrel monkey. I. Resting discharge and response to constant angular accelerations. Journal of Neurophysiology. 1971;34:635–60.

[3] Maire R, van Melle G. Diagnostic value of vestibulo-ocular reflex parameters in the detection and characterization of labyrinthine lesions. Otology & Neurotology: Official Publication of the American Otological Society, American Neurotology Society [and] European Academy of Otology and Neurotology. 2006;27:535–41. DOI: 10.1097/01.mao.0000201432.42498.08

[4] Baloh RW, Sills AW, Honrubia V. Impulsive and sinusoidal rotatory testing: a comparison with results of caloric testing. The Laryngoscope. 1979;89:646–54. DOI: 10.1288/00005537-197904000-00013

[5] Maes L, Vinck BM, Wuyts F, D'Haenens W, Bockstael A, Keppler H, Philips B, Swinnen F, Dhooge I. Clinical usefulness of the rotatory, caloric and vestibular evoked myogenic potential test in unilateral peripheral vestibular pathologies. International Journal of Audiology. 2011;50:566–76. DOI: 10.3109/14992027.2011.576706

[6] Fife TD, Tusa RJ, Furman JM, Zee DS, Frohman E, Baloh RW, Hain T, Goebel J, Demer J, Eviatar L. Assessment: vestibular testing techniques in adults and children: report of

the Therapeutics and Technology Assessment Subcommittee of the American Academy of Neurology. Neurology. 2000;55:1431–41

[7] Ahmed MF, Goebel JA, Sinks BC. Caloric test versus rotational sinusoidal harmonic acceleration and step-velocity tests in patients with and without suspected peripheral vestibulopathy. Otology & Neurotology: Official Publication of the American Otological Society, American Neurotology Society [and] European Academy of Otology and Neurotology. 2009;30:800–5. DOI: 10.1097/MAO.0b013e3181b0d02d

[8] Palomar-Asenjo V, Boleas-Aguirre MS, Sanchez-Ferrandiz N, Perez Fernandez N. Caloric and rotatory chair test results in patients with Meniere's disease. Otology & Neurotology: Official Publication of the American Otological Society, American Neurotology Society [and] European Academy of Otology and Neurotology. 2006;27:945–50. DOI: 10.1097/01.mao.0000231593.03090.23

[9] Raphan T, Matsuo V, Cohen B. Velocity storage in the vestibulo-ocular reflex arc (VOR). Experimental brain research. Experimentelle Hirnforschung. Experimentation Cerebrale. 1979;35:229–48.

[10] Laurens J, Angelaki DE. The functional significance of velocity storage and its dependence on gravity. Experimental brain research. Experimentelle Hirnforschung. Experimentation Cerebrale. 2011;210:407–22. DOI: 10.1007/s00221-011-2568-4

[11] Blair SM, Gavin M. Bainstem commissures and control of the time constant of the vestibular nystagmus. Acta Otolaryngology. 1981;91:8.

[12] Cannon JG, Demopoulos BJ, Long JP, Flynn JR, Sharabi FM. Proposed dopaminergic pharmacophore of lergotrile, pergolide and related ergot alkaloid derivatives. Journal of Medicinal Chemistry. 1981;24:238–40.

[13] Anastasio TJ. Neural network models of velocity storage in the horizontal vestibulo-ocular reflex. Biological Cybernetics. 1991;64:187–96.

[14] Galiana HL, Outerbridge JS. A bilateral model for central neural pathways in vestibuloocular reflex. Journal of Neurophysiology. 1984;51:210–41.

[15] Waespe W, Cohen B, Raphan T. Dynamic modification of the vestibulo-ocular reflex by the nodulus and uvula. Science. 1985;228:199–202.

[16] Leigh RJ, Zee DS The Neurology of Eye Movements. Oxford, New York, NY: Oxford University Press; 2006.

[17] Clarke AH, Scherer H. Caloric testing of the vestibular function during orbital flight. Adv Otorhinolaryngology. 1988;42:31–5.

[18] Scherer H, Brandt U, Clarke AH, Merbold U, Parker R. European vestibular experiments on the Spacelab-1 mission: 3. Caloric nystagmus in microgravity. Experimental brain research. Experimentelle Hirnforschung. Experimentation Cerebrale. 1986;64:255–63.

[19] Bhansali SA, Honrubia V. Current status of electronystagmography testing. Otolaryngology – Head and Neck Surgery: Official Journal of American Academy of Otolaryngology-Head and Neck Surgery. 1999;120:419–26.

[20] Rambold HA. Economic management of vertigo/dizziness disease in a county hospital: video-head-impulse test vs. caloric irrigation. European Archives of Oto-Rhino-Laryngology: Official Journal of the European Federation of Oto-Rhino-Laryngological Societies. 2015;272:2621–8. DOI: 10.1007/s00405-014-3205-1

[21] Becker GD. The screening value of monothermal caloric tests. The Laryngoscope. 1979;89:311–4. DOI: 10.1288/00005537-197902000-00015

[22] Jacobson GP, Calder JA, Shepherd VA, Rupp KA, Newman CW. Reappraisal of the monothermal warm caloric screening test. The Annals of Otology, Rhinology and Laryngology. 1995;104:942–5.

[23] Enticott JC, Dowell RC, O'Leary SJ. A comparison of the monothermal and bithermal caloric tests. Journal of Vestibular Research: Equilibrium & Orientation. 2003;13:113–9.

[24] Coats AC, Hebert F, Atwood GR. The air caloric test. A parametric study. Archives of Otolaryngology. 1976;102:343–54.

[25] Rydzewski B. A comparison of water and air stimulated bithermal-caloric test and the usefulness of both methods in otologic surgery. Otolaryngologia Polska. The Polish Otolaryngology. 2002;56:231–4.

[26] Maes L, Dhooge I, De Vel E, D'Haenens W, Bockstael A, Vinck BM. Water irrigation versus air insufflation: a comparison of two caloric test protocols. International Journal of Audiology. 2007;46:263–9. DOI: 10.1080/14992020601178147

[27] Harvey SA, Wood DJ, Feroah TR. Relationship of the head impulse test and head-shake nystagmus in reference to caloric testing. The American Journal of Otology. 1997;18:207–13.

[28] Beynon GJ, Jani P, Baguley DM. A clinical evaluation of head impulse testing. Clinical Otolaryngology and Allied Sciences. 1998;23:117–22.

[29] Weber KP, MacDougall HG, Halmagyi GM, Curthoys IS. Impulsive testing of semicircular-canal function using video-oculography. Annals of the New York Academy of Sciences. 2009;1164:486–91. DOI: 10.1111/j.1749-6632.2008.03730.x

[30] Yip CW, Glaser M, Frenzel C, Bayer O, Strupp M. Comparison of the bedside head-impulse test with the video head-impulse test in a clinical practice setting: a prospective study of 500 outpatients. Frontiers in Neurology. 2016;7:58. DOI: 10.3389/fneur.2016.00058

[31] Mahringer A, Rambold HA. Caloric test and video-head-impulse: a study of vertigo/dizziness patients in a community hospital. European Archives of Oto-Rhino-Laryng-

ology: Official Journal of the European Federation of Oto-Rhino-Laryngological Societies. 2014;271:463–72. DOI: 10.1007/s00405-013-2376-5

[32] MacDougall HG, Weber KP, McGarvie LA, Halmagyi GM, Curthoys IS. The video head impulse test: diagnostic accuracy in peripheral vestibulopathy. Neurology. 2009;73:1134–41. DOI: 10.1212/WNL.0b013e3181bacf85

[33] MacDougall HG, McGarvie LA, Halmagyi GM, Curthoys IS, Weber KP. Application of the video head impulse test to detect vertical semicircular canal dysfunction. Otology & Neurotology: Official Publication of the American Otological Society, American Neurotology Society [and] European Academy of Otology and Neurotology. 2013;34:974–9. DOI: 10.1097/MAO.0b013e31828d676d

[34] Weber KP, Aw ST, Todd MJ, McGarvie LA, Curthoys IS, Halmagyi GM. Head impulse test in unilateral vestibular loss: vestibulo-ocular reflex and catch-up saccades. Neurology. 2008;70:454–63. DOI: 10.1212/01.wnl.0000299117.48935.2e

[35] Rambold HA. Age-related refixating saccades in the three-dimensional video-head-impulse test: source and dissociation from unilateral vestibular failure. Otology & Neurotology: Official Publication of the American Otological Society, American Neurotology Society [and] European Academy of Otology and Neurotology. 2016;37:171–8. DOI: 10.1097/MAO.0000000000000947

[36] Matino-Soler E, Esteller-More E, Martin-Sanchez JC, Martinez-Sanchez JM, Perez-Fernandez N. Normative data on angular vestibulo-ocular responses in the yaw axis measured using the video head impulse test. Otology & Neurotology: Official Publication of the American Otological Society, American Neurotology Society [and] European Academy of Otology and Neurotology. 2015;36:466–71. DOI: 10.1097/MAO.0000000000000661

[37] Agrawal Y, Zuniga MG, Davalos-Bichara M, Schubert MC, Walston JD, Hughes J, Carey JP. Decline in semicircular canal and otolith function with age. Otology & Neurotology: Official Publication of the American Otological Society, American Neurotology Society [and] European Academy of Otology and Neurotology. 2012;33:832–9. DOI: 10.1097/MAO.0b013e3182545061

[38] Guerra Jimenez G, Perez Fernandez N. Reduction in posterior semicircular canal gain by age in video head impulse testing. Observational study. Acta Otorrinolaringologica Espanola. 2015. DOI: 10.1016/j.otorri.2014.12.002

[39] Mossman B, Mossman S, Purdie G, Schneider E. Age dependent normal horizontal VOR gain of head impulse test as measured with video-oculography. Journal of Otolaryngology – Head & Neck Surgery = Le Journal d'oto-rhino-laryngologie et de chirurgie cervico-faciale. 2015;44:29. DOI: 10.1186/s40463-015-0081-7

[40] McGarvie LA, MacDougall HG, Halmagyi GM, Burgess AM, Weber KP, Curthoys IS. The video head impulse test (vHIT) of semicircular canal function – age-dependent

normative values of VOR gain in healthy subjects. Frontiers in Neurology. 2015;6:154. DOI: 10.3389/fneur.2015.00154

[41] Korsager LE, Schmidt JH, Faber C, Wanscher JH. Reliability and comparison of gain values with occurrence of saccades in the EyeSeeCam video head impulse test (vHIT). European Archives of Oto-Rhino-Laryngology : Official Journal of the European Federation of Oto-Rhino-Laryngological Societies. 2016. DOI: 10.1007/s00405-016-4183-2

[42] Perez N, Rama-Lopez J. Head-impulse and caloric tests in patients with dizziness. Otology & Neurotology: Official Publication of the American Otological Society, American Neurotology Society [and] European Academy of Otology and Neurotology. 2003;24:913–7.

[43] Jorns-Haderli M, Straumann D, Palla A. Accuracy of the bedside head impulse test in detecting vestibular hypofunction. Journal of Neurology, Neurosurgery and Psychiatry. 2007;78:1113–8. DOI: 10.1136/jnnp.2006.109512

[44] Scherer H, Clarke AH. The caloric vestibular reaction in space. Physiological considerations. Acta Oto-Laryngologica. 1985;100:328–36.

[45] Haque A, Angelaki DE, Dickman JD. Spatial tuning and dynamics of vestibular semicircular canal afferents in rhesus monkeys. Experimental brain research. Experimentelle Hirnforschung. Experimentation Cerebrale. 2004;155:81–90. DOI: 10.1007/s00221-003-1693-0

[46] Goldberg JM. Afferent diversity and the organization of central vestibular pathways. Experimental brain research. Experimentelle Hirnforschung. Experimentation Cerebrale. 2000;130:277–97.

[47] McGarvie LA, Curthoys IS, MacDougall HG, Halmagyi GM. What does the dissociation between the results of video head impulse versus caloric testing reveal about the vestibular dysfunction in Meniere's disease? Acta Oto-Laryngologica. 2015;135:859–65. DOI: 10.3109/00016489.2015.1015606

[48] Bartolomeo M, Biboulet R, Pierre G, Mondain M, Uziel A, Venail F. Value of the video head impulse test in assessing vestibular deficits following vestibular neuritis. European Archives of Oto-Rhino-Laryngology: Official Journal of the European Federation of Oto-Rhino-Laryngological Societies. 2013. DOI: 10.1007/s00405-013-2451

[49] Redondo-Martinez J, Becares-Martinez C, Orts-Alborch M, Garcia-Callejo FJ, Perez-Carbonell T, Marco-Algarra J. Relationship between video head impulse test (vHIT) and caloric test in patients with vestibular neuritis. Acta Otorrinolaringologica Espanola. 2016;67:156–61. DOI: 10.1016/j.otorri.2015.07.005

[50] Zellhuber S, Mahringer A, Rambold HA. Relation of video-head-impulse test and caloric irrigation: a study on the recovery in unilateral vestibular neuritis. European Archives of Oto-Rhino-Laryngology: Official Journal of the European Federation of

Oto-Rhino-Laryngological Societies. 2014;271:2375–83. DOI: 10.1007/s00405-013-2723-6

[51] Schmid-Priscoveanu A, Bohmer A, Obzina H, Straumann D. Caloric and search-coil head-impulse testing in patients after vestibular neuritis. Journal of the Association for Research in Otolaryngology. 2001;2:72–8.

[52] Manzari L, Burgess AM, MacDougall HG, Curthoys IS. Vestibular function after vestibular neuritis. International Journal of Audiology. 2013;52:713–8. DOI: 10.3109/14992027.2013.809485

[53] Zhang D, Fan Z, Han Y, Yu G, Wang H. Inferior vestibular neuritis: a novel subtype of vestibular neuritis. The Journal of Laryngology and Otology. 2010;124:477–81. DOI: 10.1017/S0022215109992337

[54] Chihara Y, Iwasaki S, Murofushi T, Yagi M, Inoue A, Fujimoto C, Egami N, Ushio M, Karino S, Sugasawa K, Yamasoba T. Clinical characteristics of inferior vestibular neuritis. Acta Oto-Laryngologica. 2012;132:1288–94. DOI: 10.3109/00016489.2012.701326

[55] Kim JS, Kim HJ. Inferior vestibular neuritis. Journal of Neurology. 2012;259:1553–60. DOI: 10.1007/s00415-011-6375-4

[56] Rambold HA. Prediction of short-term outcome in acute superior vestibular nerve failure: three-dimensional video-head-impulse test and caloric irrigation. International Journal of Otolaryngology. 2015;2015:639024. DOI: 10.1155/2015/639024

[57] Lee SU, Kim HJ, Koo JW, Kim JS. Comparison of caloric and head-impulse tests during the attacks of Meniere's disease. The Laryngoscope. 2016. DOI: 10.1002/lary.26103

[58] Blodow A, Heinze M, Bloching MB, von Brevern M, Radtke A, Lempert T. Caloric stimulation and video-head impulse testing in Meniere's disease and vestibular migraine. Acta Oto-Laryngologica. 2014;134:1239–44. DOI: 10.3109/00016489.2014.939300

[59] Manzari L, MacDougall HG, Burgess AM, Curthoys IS. New, fast, clinical vestibular tests identify whether a vertigo attack is due to early Meniere's disease or vestibular neuritis. The Laryngoscope. 2013;123:507–11. DOI: 10.1002/lary.23479

[60] Zulueta-Santos C, Lujan B, Manrique-Huarte R, Perez-Fernandez N. The vestibulo-ocular reflex assessment in patients with Meniere's disease: examining all semicircular canals. Acta Oto-Laryngologica. 2014;134:1128–33. DOI: 10.3109/00016489.2014.919405

[61] von Brevern M, Neuhauser H. Epidemiological evidence for a link between vertigo and migraine. Journal of Vestibular Research: Equilibrium & Orientation. 2011;21:299–304. DOI: 10.3233/VES-2011-0423

[62] Neugebauer H, Adrion C, Glaser M, Strupp M. Long-term changes of central ocular motor signs in patients with vestibular migraine. European Neurology. 2013;69:102–7. DOI: 10.1159/000343814

[63] Yollu U, Uluduz DU, Yilmaz M, Yener HM, Akil F, Kuzu B, Kara E, Hayir D, Ceylan D, Korkut N. Vestibular migraine screening in a migraine-diagnosed patient population and assessment of vestibulocochlear function. Clinical Otolaryngology: Official Journal of ENT-UK; Official Journal of Netherlands Society for Oto-Rhino-Laryngology & Cervico-Facial Surgery. 2016. DOI: 10.1111/coa.12699

[64] Lee JW, Jung JY, Chung YS, Suh MW. Clinical manifestation and prognosis of vestibular migraine according to the vestibular function test results. Korean Journal of Audiology. 2013;17:18–22. DOI: 10.7874/kja.2013.17.1.18

[65] Foster CA, Pollard CK. Comparison of caloric reactivity between migraineurs and non-migraineurs. The Journal of Laryngology and Otology. 2015;129:960–3. DOI: 10.1017/S0022215115002066

[66] Yang Y, Zhuang J, Zhou L, Tong B, Zhou X, Gao B. Comparison of caloric responses between vestibular migraine and Meniere disease patients. Lin chuang er bi yan hou tou jing wai ke za zhi = Journal of Clinical Otorhinolaryngology, Head and Neck Surgery. 2016;30:15–8.

[67] Boldingh MI, Ljostad U, Mygland A, Monstad P. Comparison of interictal vestibular function in vestibular migraine vs migraine without vertigo. Headache. 2013;53:1123–33. DOI: 10.1111/head.12129

[68] Andersen JF, Nilsen KS, Vassbotn FS, Moller P, Myrseth E, Lund-Johansen M, Goplen FK. Predictors of vertigo in patients with untreated vestibular schwannoma. Otology & Neurotology: Official Publication of the American Otological Society, American Neurotology Society [and] European Academy of Otology and Neurotology. 2015;36:647–52. DOI: 10.1097/MAO.0000000000000668

[69] Machner B, Gottschalk S, Sander T, Helmchen C, Rambold H. Intralabyrinthine schwannoma affecting the low but not high frequency function of the vestibulo-ocular reflex: implications for the clinical diagnosis of chronic peripheral vestibular deficits. Journal of Neurology, Neurosurgery and Psychiatry. 2007;78:772–4. DOI: 10.1136/jnnp.2006.106179

[70] Blodow A, Helbig R, Wichmann N, Wenzel A, Walther LE, Bloching MB. Video head impulse test or caloric irrigation?. Contemporary diagnostic tests for vestibular schwannoma. HNO. 2013;61:781–5. DOI: 10.1007/s00106-013-2752-x

[71] Tranter-Entwistle I, Dawes P, Darlington CL, Smith PF, Cutfield N. Video head impulse in comparison to caloric testing in unilateral vestibular schwannoma. Acta Oto-Laryngologica. 2016;136(11):1110–1114

[72] Tringali S, Charpiot A, Ould MB, Dubreuil C, Ferber-Viart C. Characteristics of 629 vestibular schwannomas according to preoperative caloric responses. Otology & Neurotology: Official Publication of the American Otological Society, American Neurotology Society [and] European Academy of Otology and Neurotology. 2010;31:467–72. DOI: 10.1097/MAO.0b013e3181cdd8b7

[73] Suzuki M, Yamada C, Inoue R, Kashio A, Saito Y, Nakanishi W. Analysis of vestibular testing in patients with vestibular schwannoma based on the nerve of origin, the localization and the size of the tumor. Otology & Neurotology: Official Publication of the American Otological Society, American Neurotology Society [and] European Academy of Otology and Neurotology. 2008;29:1029–33. DOI: 10.1097/MAO.0b013e3181845854

[74] Taylor RL, Kong J, Flanagan S, Pogson J, Croxson G, Pohl D, Welgampola MS. Prevalence of vestibular dysfunction in patients with vestibular schwannoma using video head-impulses and vestibular-evoked potentials. Journal of Neurology. 2015;262:1228–37. DOI: 10.1007/s00415-015-7697-4

[75] Rambold H, Boenki J, Stritzke G, Wisst F, Neppert B, Helmchen C. Differential vestibular dysfunction in sudden unilateral hearing loss. Neurology. 2005;64:148–51. DOI: 10.1212/01.WNL.0000148599.18397.D2

[76] Pogson JM, Taylor RL, Young AS, McGarvie LA, Flanagan S, Halmagyi GM, Welgampola MS. Vertigo with sudden hearing loss: audio-vestibular characteristics. Journal of Neurology. 2016;263(10):2086–96. DOI: 10.1007/s00415-016-8214-0

[77] Kim S, Oh YM, Koo JW, Kim JS. Bilateral vestibulopathy: clinical characteristics and diagnostic criteria. Otology & Neurotology: Official Publication of the American Otological Society, American Neurotology Society [and] European Academy of Otology and Neurotology. 2011;32:812–7. DOI: 10.1097/MAO.0b013e31821a3b7d

[78] Weber KP, Aw ST, Todd MJ, McGarvie LA, Curthoys IS, Halmagyi GM. Horizontal head impulse test detects gentamicin vestibulotoxicity. Neurology. 2009;72:1417–24. DOI: 10.1212/WNL.0b013e3181a18652

[79] Moon M, Chang SO, Kim MB. Diverse clinical and laboratory manifestations of bilateral vestibulopathy. The Laryngoscope. 2016.Epub. DOI: 10.1002/lary.25946

[80] Fujimoto C, Kinoshita M, Kamogashira T, Egami N, Sugasawa K, Yamasoba T, Iwasaki S. Characteristics of vertigo and the affected vestibular nerve systems in idiopathic bilateral vestibulopathy. Acta Oto-Laryngologica. 2016;136:43–7. DOI: 10.3109/00016489.2015.1082193

[81] Tarnutzer AA, Bockisch CJ, Buffone E, Weiler S, Bachmann LM, Weber KP. Disease-specific sparing of the anterior semicircular canals in bilateral vestibulopathy. Clinical Neurophysiology: Official Journal of the International Federation of Clinical Neurophysiology. 2016;127:2791–801. DOI: 10.1016/j.clinph.2016.05.005

[82] Szmulewicz DJ, McLean CA, MacDougall HG, Roberts L, Storey E, Halmagyi GM. CANVAS an update: clinical presentation, investigation and management. Journal of Vestibular Research: Equilibrium & Orientation. 2014;24:465–74. DOI: 10.3233/VES-140536

[83] Kattah JC, Talkad AV, Wang DZ, Hsieh YH, Newman-Toker DE. HINTS to diagnose stroke in the acute vestibular syndrome: three-step bedside oculomotor examination

more sensitive than early MRI diffusion-weighted imaging. Stroke. 2009;40:3504–10. DOI: 10.1161/STROKEAHA.109.551234

[84] Mantokoudis G, Tehrani AS, Wozniak A, Eibenberger K, Kattah JC, Guede CI, Zee DS, Newman-Toker DE. VOR gain by head impulse video-oculography differentiates acute vestibular neuritis from stroke. Otology & Neurotology: Official Publication of the American Otological Society, American Neurotology Society [and] European Academy of Otology and Neurotology. 2015;36:457–65. DOI: 10.1097/MAO.0000000000000638

[85] Newman-Toker DE, Saber Tehrani AS, Mantokoudis G, Pula JH, Guede CI, Kerber KA, Blitz A, Ying SH, Hsieh YH, Rothman RE, Hanley DF, Zee DS, Kattah JC. Quantitative video-oculography to help diagnose stroke in acute vertigo and dizziness: toward an ECG for the eyes. Stroke. 2013;44:1158–61. DOI: 10.1161/STROKEAHA.111.000033

[86] Choi KD, Lee H, Kim JS. Ischemic syndromes causing dizziness and vertigo. Handbook of Clinical Neurology. 2016;137:317–40. DOI: 10.1016/B978-0-444-63437-5.00023-6

Chapter 10

OAEs and Meniere Disease

Stavros Hatzopoulos, Andrea Ciorba,
Virginia Corazzi and Piotr Henryk Skarzynski

Additional information is available at the end of the chapter

http://dx.doi.org/10.5772/66387

Abstract

Otoacoustic emissions (OAEs) are responses originating from the inner ear. Clinically they are evoked by different families of acoustic stimuli, such as transient acoustic clicks, tone pips, and pure tones. Upon stimulation, the acoustic energy is transformed in the middle ear at acoustic pressure acting upon the stapes footplate. The pressure wave inside the cochlea stimulates the OAE generators and a reverse acoustic energy (the OAE response) propagates from the inner ear, through the stapes and the middle ear structures, to the tympanic membrane. Considering that the acoustic energy has to cross the middle ear structures twice, the functional status of the middle ear can influence or attenuate considerably the OAE response. In this context, any vestibular alteration can influence the middle ear mechanics (mainly the middle ear impedance) and consequently the OAE response characteristics. The data in the literature indicate that OAEs are very sensitive to changes in the intracranial pressure. These pressure alterations during the Meniere's hydrops phase are expressed as changes in the intralabyrinthine pressure. Other studies have presented data supporting the assumption that OAEs can adequately monitor middle ear changes induced by the presentation of the glycerol test. The data in the literature suggest that OAEs can monitor the progress of Meniere's disease using reliable indices.

Keywords: Ménière, hearing threshold, glycerol test, vestibule, otoacoustic emissions, distortion product otoacoustic emissions, transient otoacoustic emissions, middle ear mechanics

1. Introduction

Otoacoustic emissions (OAEs) are responses originating from the inner ear and they were first described by David Kemp [1, 2]. They are evoked by different families of acoustic stimuli, such as transient acoustic clicks and chirps, tone pips, and pure tones. Upon stimulation, the

INTECH
open science | open minds

© 2017 The Author(s). Licensee InTech. This chapter is distributed under the terms of the Creative Commons Attribution License (http://creativecommons.org/licenses/by/3.0), which permits unrestricted use, distribution, and reproduction in any medium, provided the original work is properly cited. (cc) BY

acoustic energy is transformed by the middle ear in acoustic pressure applied to the stapes footplate. The pressure wave inside the cochlea stimulates the OAE generators and a reverse acoustic energy (the OAE response) propagates from the inner ear, through the stapes and the middle ear structures, to the tympanic membrane. There it can be recorded by a sensitive probe (microphone), inserted in the acoustic meatus.

The classical classification scheme categorizes OAEs according to their evoking stimulus [3]. In this context, the OAE responses can be elicited by transient clicks (TEOAEs), transient tone bursts (TBOAEs), or by pure tones (distortion product OAEs – DPOAEs). Responses evoked by random thermal noise in the cochlea are called Spontaneous OAEs (SOAEs), which have limited clinical applications. The newest and most accepted taxonomy classifies the responses according to their generation mechanisms [4]. According to Shera and Guinnan [4], the OAE responses are evoked by a linear reflection (of the travelling wave energy) on the basilar membrane, or by nonlinear processes "orchestrated" by nonlinear characteristics of the outer hair cells (OHCs) and the cochlear amplifier per se. The clinically used responses (TEOAEs or DPOAEs) are a mixture of these two mechanisms.

The OAE values, express a measure/metric of the cochlear amplifier functionality, which has found numerous applications in Audiology and Hearing Science. The most known application is in the area of hearing screening. TEOAEs can detect sensorineural deficits up to 35 dB HL; DPOAEs are more sensitive and can detect deficits up to 40 dB HL [3]. The great advantage of OAEs, in comparison to traditional audiometry tests, is that they can detect a deficit before it registers as a hearing deficit (i.e., it is in a subclinical phase) [3]. When an external or internal stressor causes severe mechanical alterations on the functionality of the OHCs, intrinsic and extrinsic apoptotic processes are initiated [5]. Within the next time-frames (days/months), the corresponding OAEs are severely altered and gradually, the OHC damage induces an intrinsic neural apoptosis and a subsequent hearing deficit.

Therefore, the OAE response characteristics are altered by inner ear disorders, such as Meniere's disease (MD), a condition in which the whole inner ear can be damaged, including all the structures of the cochlea (outer and inner hair cells) and the vestibular system.

This chapter is an excursus of the current scientific findings relating vestibular and middle ear alterations, as observed in various stages of the Ménière's disease, with measurements of otoacoustic emissions. The latter are considered the test of choice to identify preclinical effects on the human hearing threshold and alterations in the inner ear.

2. A short introduction of Ménière's disease (MD)

MD is an idiopathic disorder of the inner ear. It is characterized by paroxysmal unpredictable crisis, with a typical symptomatological triad: tinnitus, hearing loss associated to fullness and objective vertigo with neurovegetative symptoms [6]. The crises have a variable duration (from few minutes to 24 h) and the intercritical periods are characterized by residual dizziness or wellness, configuring, anyway, a particularly invalidating disease, particularly considering the unpredictability of the crisis.

MD occurs typically between the fourth and sixth decades of life, with a mild prevalence in women. It is frequently unilateral, but both ears may be affected with the progression of the disease. Although most cases of MD are sporadic, a 5-15% has a familiar configuration and seems to have a hereditary transmission.

To date, the etiology of MD is unknown, but anatomopathological and histopathological studies on Menieric patients temporal bones, have revealed an enlargement of the membranous labyrinth due to an endolymphatic hydrops [7, 8]. Therefore, the most accredited theory about MD pathogenetic mechanism is the increase of the endolymphatic volume, due to a disorder of either production or reabsorption mechanisms of endolymph, with an expansion and a possible rupture of the membranous labyrinth [9–11]. The damage to the hair cells may be due to both the pressure, during the hydrops phase, and the mixture of endolymph and perilymph, if the membrane rupture occurs. In this case particularly, it has been stated that the crisis may be produced by a potassium intoxication of the labyrinth sensorial epithelium, after the Reissner's membrane rupture [12, 13].

Even though infrequent, endolymphatic hydrops can be congenital and it may be consequent to inner ear malformations, such as Mondini dysplasia [14]. More frequently, the acquired hydrops can be a consequence of viral or bacterial labyrinth infections, or traumas [15].

It has been reported that endolymphatic hydrops has been observed also in asymptomatic patients; this suggests that there should be many 'triggering factors' that may rouse a MD crisis, such as hydric retention, viral infections, stress, cranial traumas, vitamin deficiency, and endocrine disorders [16].

The diagnosis of MD is difficult and it can be defined only after some vestibular crisis with the typical triad. In 1995, the American Academy of Otolaryngology-Head and Neck Surgery published the diagnostic criteria for MD, then updated in 2015, defining a "possible", "probable", and "definite" MD, depending on the frequency of the typical symptoms, until the "confirmed" diagnosis of MD, achievable only with a histopathological examination [17, 18]. A careful history taking and the audiovestibular instrumental examination are recommended. Otoscopy is usually negative.

In the initial phases of MD, the tonal audiometry finds a unilateral cochlear sensorineural hearing loss, affecting the low frequencies. At the beginning, the MD hearing loss is typically fluctuating, reflecting the inner ear hydrops phase: only during this phase, it is possible to perform an osmotic test (Glycerol test) and to observe the improvement of 10 dB in the hearing threshold, at least on two frequencies between 500 Hz and 2000 Hz, within 3 hours, after the administration of 1.5 ml/Kg of body weight of oral glycerol (a potent osmotic agent) with the same volume of isotonic saline solution [19, 20]. The glycerol test is not a diagnostic evaluation, but it allows in determining the reversibility of the early phase of MD and, therefore, it has a prognostic and therapeutic significance. The verbal discrimination is initially preserved at the vocal audiometry. In an advanced MD, hearing loss becomes permanent, pantonal, and often bilateral [21, 22]. The evaluation of the acoustic reflex threshold also demonstrates the recruitment phenomenon, typical of cochlear lesions. Auditory brainstem responses (ABR) can exclude a retrocochlear disease. The vestibular instrumental examinations could be normal at the beginning; during the progress of MD, it reveals a unilateral vestibular hyporeflectivity. Electrocochleography can determine, during the hydropic phase, an increased summating potential, due to the distension of basilar membrane into the scala tympani and then an increased action potential/summating potential ratio [23].

Neuroimaging, such as laboratory exams, are recommended during the differential diagnosis in order to exclude other diseases causing Ménière's-like symptoms or congenital malformation/anatomic variations of the inner ear or metabolic, electrolytic, endocrine, vitaminic, immunologic disorders potentially implicated in MD [24].

3. OAEs and MD

It has been suggested that OAEs and, in particular, distortion product otoacoustic emissions (DPOAEs), may determine the important information about which cochlear regions have been involved in the first phase of MD characterized by recurrent hydropic crisis [25, 26]. Considering that the acoustic energy has to cross the middle ear structures twice, OAE response may be reduced or even suppressed due to imperfections of the middle ear transmission mechanism. In this context, inner ear disorders can influence the OAE response characteristics [27]. The endolymphatic hydrops (confined primarily in the cochlear duct and in the saccule [15]), increase the impedance at the level of the stapes, attenuating any forward or backward acoustic energy transmissions [28].

4. DPOAEs and MD

De Kleine et al. [29] found that, in patients affected by MD, DPOAEs have smaller amplitude than the unaffected ears in relation to the mechanical alterations which were hydrops-induced. An early report on MD by Eggermont and Schmidt [30] stated that in the early phase of MD, a minimal variation on the outer hairy cells function, caused by hydrops, can determine the typical auditory threshold fluctuation; this phenomenon can be indirectly observed as a reduction in the DPOAE amplitude particularly in the low DPOAE frequencies. In cases of advanced MD, the severe damage or the loss of inner ear, outer hair cells, is responsible for DPOAEs absence. Unfortunately, these claims have not been verified in subsequent reports and one of the criticisms Eggermont received [31] was that DPOAEs have very low signal-to-noise ratios (S/N) at the lower frequencies (i.e., 0.5 kHz and 0.75 kHz).

DPOAEs have also been considered as an objective monitor system, for any middle ear functional changes induced by the administration of the glycerol test [32], during the hydrops phase of MD. The osmotic effect and its influence on the intracranial pressure determine a reduction of the labyrinth hypertension, because of the movements of fluids outside the inner ear. This effect can be monitored through: (i) a tonal/vocal audiometry. Effects include a hearing threshold improvement of 10 dB HL in least two frequencies between 500 Hz and 2000 Hz, or an improvement of the verbal intelligibility score of at least 10%; (ii) through electrocochleography (EchoG). Effects include a decrease of the summating potential amplitude [33]; (iii) through OAEs, in particular with an improvement of the DPOAEs amplitude [19]. Overall, the data in the literature [19, 20, 29, 32] suggest that DPOAEs can monitor successfully how glycerol recovers the hearing threshold, compromised by the presence of hydrops.

DPOAEs are very sensitive to changes in the intracranial pressure [34]. Although Rotter et al. [35] found that DPOAEs are not as accurate as the transtympanic electrocochleography, other authors [27, 29, 30] support the role of DPOAEs as a reliable method allowing the detection of endolymphatic hydrops and the cochlear damage in MD [19, 33].

Theoretically, an MD case presenting multiple lesions in the inner ear should condition the OAE responses. In this context, one expects that the OAE responses should be attenuated at low or at high frequencies. There are a few reports in the literature showing the exact opposite [36]. In a study by van Huffelen et al. [36], MD cases were classified into 4 groups. When hearing thresholds were above 60 dB HL, no detectable OAEs were recorded. For those cases, presenting hearing thresholds within 30–60 dB HL, abnormally high DPOAE responses were observed. The authors suggested that these emissions are generated by cochlear sites, sustaining the residual hearing of the patient. Some MD case studies have also been reported presenting anomalous DPOAEs. Hall [37] describes a case diagnosed with a unilateral MD, where the left ear DPOAE responses were shown to be quite robust, despite the fact that the audiogram showed a low-frequency sensorineural hearing impairment. The same author shows that data analyses from groups of MD patients follow the patterns reported widely in the literature (i.e., attenuation of OAEs caused by OHC dysfunction).

5. TEOAEs and MD

One of the first publications relating MD with TEOAEs was a German study by Nubel et al [38]. Their data supported the hypothesis that a combination of TEOAEs and a masker tone at 30 Hz (in an adjustable relation to one another) could discriminate well cases of endolymphatic hydrops. Their protocol examines TEOAE suppression at 0° and 270°. For the latter, normal subjects showed a complete suppression, whereas MD cases showed partial or no suppression. The same protocol was reevaluated in a subsequent study by Hof-Duin and Wit [39], who reported that the Nubel et al. model was correct but their interpretation of the data was erroneous. According to Hof-Duin and Wit, the observed changes were not directly caused by the endolymphatic hydrops but by other alterations in inner ear structures, for example, in the gain of the cochlear amplifier (i.e., induced hearing loss).

The search for a particular TEOAE pattern in MD patients has not been very successful. TEOAEs detect alterations in the middle ear stimulus transmission or in the stimulus decodification and amplification (cochlea). From a TEOAE point of view, MD cases presenting hearing losses are identical to cases presenting a sensorineural deficit. **Figures 1** and **2** present TEOAE data obtained from the two subjects presenting an initial phase MD. The characteristics of these cases were similar: no use of drugs and prolonged exposure to noise, a low frequency humming feeling (tinnitus), and dizziness. Pure tone audiometry revealed a moderate hearing loss in the low frequencies up to 1.0 kHz. Acoustic Immitance and stapedial reflexes were found normal. Subject 1 was a female of 46 years old. Subject 2 was a male of 37 years old. The TEOAE responses indicate a sensorineural deficit and are **indistinguishable** from other responses originating from patients with sensorineural deficits.

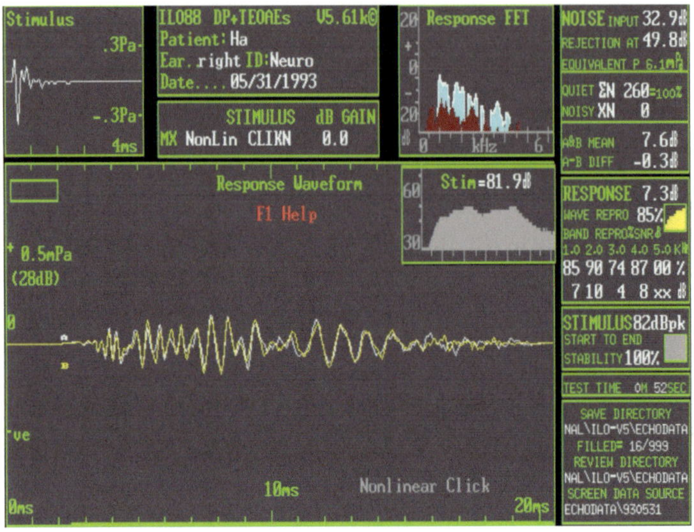

Figure 1. Subject 1: female 46 years, with a typical MD hearing loss profile. Pure tone audiometry revealed a moderate hearing loss, in low frequencies. The TEOAE S/N ratios indicate responses up to 4 kHz, an indication of a normally functioning (although partially compromised) cochlea.

Hatzopoulos et al. [40] used advanced time-frequency (TF) spectral methods to examine the frequency content of TEOAE responses from patients presenting sensorineural deficits. Forty subjects presenting moderate hearing losses (in the range of 1.0 kHz to 8.0 kHz) were enrolled in the study. Five of these subjects were MD cases (two of them are presented in **Figures 1** and **2**). The TF patterns from these subjects followed the TF profiles of the other sensorineural cases and no particular TF-markers were observed for the MD subgroup.

TEOAEs have been employed in the detection of the hearing impairment component of MD. A French group, coordinated by Paul Avan, has made considerable contributions to the influence of intralabyrinthine pressure and endolymphatic hydrops on evoked emissions [25, 28, 41–43]. One way to understand this influence is to assess the alterations of the TEOAE phase shift (the latter is a component provided by the FFT decomposition of the TEOAE response). According to Mom et al. [41], "Acoustic phase shift highlights a variation in intra-cochlear functioning that is worth understanding. By analogy to what is observed in intracranial pressure variation as described by Büki et al. [42], it is logical to expect a marked disturbance in intralabyrinthine pressure. There may be a change in the rigidity of the annular ligament of the footplate under pressure from the perilymphatic compartment that is pushed back by the endolymphatic compartment containing the hydrops; or there may be some more subtle endocochlear modification. The endocochlear pressure resulting from change of posture would be the equivalent for the "hydropic" cochlea of a considerable rise in intracranial pressure. In Büki et al.'s experiment, the functioning of a normal cochlea reflected change in intracranial pressure [42]. In MD, however, cochlear functioning is not normal, by definition. As the model does not distinguish which part of the inner ear is being measured but considers it as a single whole, it can reasonably be considered applicable even in a pathological ear. TEOAE phase change in a test performed in an ear affected by MD during the acute phase may be attributed to the hair bundle of the outer hair cells (OHCs). OHC hair bundle inclination,

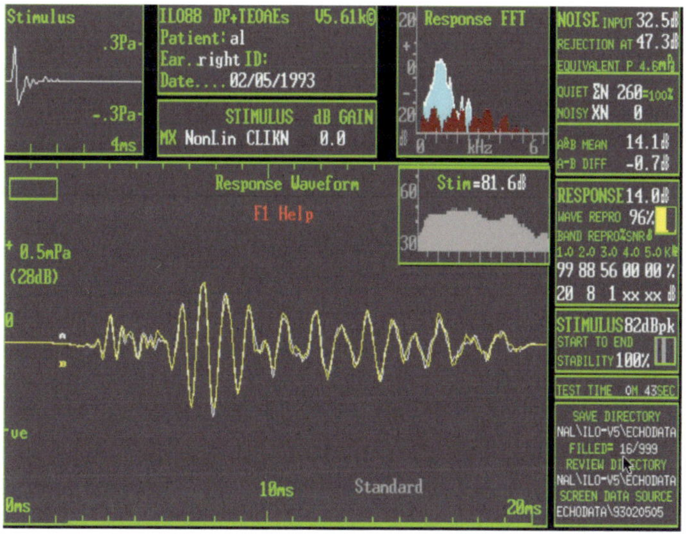

Figure 2. Subject 2: male 37 years, with a typical MD hearing loss profile. Pure tone audiometry revealed a mild to moderate hearing loss, in the low frequencies. The majority of the TEOAE energy is concentrated around 1–1.5 kHz. The TEOAE S/N ratios above 3.0 kHz indicate lack of responses. How this response can be possible, when the pure tone audiometry shows a low frequency deficit? Most probably the strong TEOAE response (from the first 6–10 ms in the TEOAE trace) is generated by cochlear regions above 1.0 kHz, where the subject presents better hearing thresholds.

inducing opening of specific ion channels, compared to gating springs, determines OHC excitation level, which in turn defines the OHC resting point which may shift along the characteristic OHC input-output (I-O) curve, as faithfully reflected in the amplitudes of some types of OAE (quadratic distortion-product OAEs) or in the phase of others. The data from Büki et al showed that phase shift was significantly elevated beyond the normal interval in 18 of the MD patients with range, –80° to +145° and sensitivity, 90%. Overall, in patients, in whom the transient evoked OAEs (TEOAEs) were present, positive predictive value was 100% and negative predictive value was 92.3%.

Two different groups in Japan have assessed the effects of the glycerol test on the TEOAE variables, and have reported different success rates. In the study by Inoue et al. [44] two groups were assessed: one classified as Meniere (22 ears) and one as Meniere with cochlear losses (20 ears). Three hours after a 1.5 g/kg glycerol administration, patients from both groups were assessed with TEOAEs and pure tone audiometry. The authors report that the TEOAE evocation rate (i.e., identification of a robust TEOAE response) improved in both groups: in the MD group from 50% to 63.6% and in the cochlear MD group from 66.7% to 83.3%. The findings from Sakashita paper [45] are different. The glycerol effect on TEOAEs was decomposed on the effects on four aspects of the TEOAE waveform, including the "Total TEOAE Response Power", or the "Filtered TEOAE response power" in the 1–2.0 kHz range. They reported positive results in 11/22 ears and added that positive TEOAE results were present independently of the threshold improvement in the 1.0 and 2.0 kHz octaves. Interestingly they reported that a DPOAE protocol (a DPOAE growth function at 1.0, 1.5, 2.0 kHz) was more sensitive to the glycerol test. They concluded that the DPOAE values at 1.0 and 1.5 kHz are useful for a clinical practice.

6. Conclusions

The data in the literature suggest that OAEs represent a valid noninvasive instrument, which can monitor the cochlear damage entity in patients affected by MD, and could also monitor its progress. OAEs are not just reliable tools, but they are a low-cost methodology in comparison to standardized MD monitoring methods, such as electrocochleography.

The data in the literature shows that alterations in the inner ear caused by the presence of a hydrops can be monitored accurately with OAEs. Glycerol results can also be monitored successfully. Some reports suggest that a DPOAE protocol can be more suitable for MD monitoring tasks, but considering the mechanisms of OAE generation this might not be true. TEOAEs and DPOAEs can similarly detect inner ear alterations as long as these affect the basilar membrane mobility and the functioning of outer hair cells.

Although promising, this field of research still needs to be expanded, where experimental studies are lacking. It is likely that in the future, either implementing our knowledge among MD, or implementing the OAE technology, the application of the OAE for patients affected by MD could be further expanded and offered with more information to the clinical practice.

Acknowledgements

This work was supported by the project "Integrated system of tools for diagnostics and telerehabilitation of sensory organs disorders (hearing, vision, speech, balance, taste, smell)" acr. INNOSNESE, co-financed by the National Centre for Research and Development (Poland), within the STRATEGMED program.

Author details

Stavros Hatzopoulos[1*], Andrea Ciorba[1], Virginia Corazzi[1] and Piotr Henryk Skarzynski[2, 3, 4]

*Address all correspondence to: sdh1@unife.it

1 ENT & Audiology Department, University Hospital of Ferrara, Ferrara, Italy

2 World Hearing Center, Warsaw, Poland

3 Department of Heart Failure and Cardiac Rehabilitation, Medical University of Warsaw, Warsaw, Poland

4 Institute of Sensory Organs, Kajetany, Poland

References

[1] Kemp DT. Stimulated acoustic emissions from within the human auditory system. *J Acoust Soc Am* 1978;64(5):1386-1391.

[2] Kemp DT. The evoked cochlear mechanical response and the auditory microstructure – evidence for a new element in cochlear mechanics. *Scand Audiol Suppl* 1979;(9):35-47.

[3] Probst R, Lonsbury-Martin BL, Martin GK. A review of otoacoustic emissions. *J Acoust Soc Am* 1991;89(5):2027-2067.

[4] Shera CA, Guinan JJ Jr. Evoked otoacoustic emissions arise by two fundamentally different mechanisms: a taxonomy for mammalian OAEs. *J Acoust Soc Am* 1999;105(2 Pt 1):782-798.

[5] Furness DN. Molecular basis of hair cell loss. *Cell Tissue Res* 2015; 361(1) 387-399.

[6] Enander A, Stahle J. Hearing in Ménière's disease. *Acta Oto-Laryng* 1967;64:543-556.

[7] Hallpike C, Cairns H. Observations on the pathology of Ménière's syndrome. *J Laryngol Otol* 1938;53:625-655.

[8] Schmidt PH Jr., Brunsting RC, Antvelink JB. Ménière's disease: etiology and natural history. *Acta Otolaryngol* 1979;87:410-412.

[9] Horner KC. Functional changes associated with experimentally induced endolymphatic hydrops. *Hear Res* 1993;68:1-18.

[10] Takeuchi S, Takeda T, Saito H. Pressure relationship between perilymph and endolymph associated with endolymphatic infusion. *Ann Otol Rhinol Laryngol* 1991;100:244-248.

[11] Wit HP, Warmerdam TJ, Albers FWJ. Measurement of the mechanical compliance of the endolymphatic compartments in the guinea pig. *Hear Res* 2000;145:82-90.

[12] Rauch S, Merchant SN, Thedinger BA. Meniere's syndrome and endolymphatic hydrops. Double-blind temporal bone study. *Ann Otol Rhinol Laryngol* 1989;98:873-883.

[13] Antoli-Candela F. The histopathology of Meniere's disease. *Acta Otolaryngol* 1976;340(suppl):1-42.

[14] Schuknecht HF. Mondini dysplasia. A clinical pathophysiological study. *Ann Otol Rhinol Laryngol* 1980;89(suppl);1-23.

[15] Schuknecht HF, Gulya AJ. Endolymphatic hydrops. An overview and classification. *Ann Otol Rhinol Laryngol Suppl* 1983, 106:1-20.

[16] Paparella MM. Pathogenesis and pathophysiology of Meniere's disease. *Acta Otolaryngol Suppl* 1991;485:26-35.

[17] Committee on hearing and equilibrium. Guidelines for the diagnosis and evaluation of therapy in Meniere's disease. *Otolaryngol Head Neck Surg* 1995;113:181-185.

[18] Lopez-Escamez JA, Carey J, Chung WH, Goebel JA, Magnusson M, Mandalà M, Newman-Toker DE, Strupp M, Suzuki M, Trabalzini F, Bisdorff A; Classification Committee of the Barany Society; Japan Society for Equilibrium Research; European Academy of Otology and Neurotology (EAONO); Equilibrium Committee of the American Academy of Otolaryngology-Head and Neck Surgery (AAO-HNS); Korean Balance Society. Diagnostic criteria for Menière's disease. *J Vestib Res*. 2015;25(1):1-7.

[19] Jablonka-Strom A, Pospiech L, Zatonski M, Bochnia M. Dynamics of pure tone audiometry and DPOAE changes induced by glycerol in Meniere's disease. *Eur Arch Otorhinolaryngol* 2013;270(5):1751-1756.

[20] Basel T, Lutkenhoner B. Auditory threshold shifts after glycerol administration to patients with suspected Meniere's disease: a retrospective analysis. *Ear Hear* 2013;34(3):370-384.

[21] Morrison AW. Predictive tests for Meniere's disease. *Am J Otol* 1986;7:5-10.

[22] Friberg L, Stahle J, Svedberg A. The natural course of Ménière's disease. *Acta Otolaryngol (Stockh)* 1984;406(suppl):72-77.

[23] Horst JW, De Kleine E. Audiogram fine structure and spontaneous otoacoustic emissions in patients with Meniere's disease. *Audiology* 1999;38:267-270.

[24] Hamann KF, Arnold W. Meniere's disease. *Adv Otorhinolaryngol* 1999;55:137-168.

[25] Harris FP, Probst R. Transiently evoked otoacoustic emissions in patients with Meniere's disease. *Acta Otolaryngol (Stockh)* 1992;112:36-44.

[26] van Huffelen WM, Mateijsen DJM, Wit HP. Classification of patient with Meniere's disease using otoacoustic emissions. *Audiol Neurootol* 1998;3:419-430.

[27] Avan P, Durrant JD, Buki B. Possible effects of cochlear hydrops and related phenomena on OAEs. *Sem Hear* 2001;22:405-414.

[28] Avan P, Giraudet F, Chauveau B, Gilain L, Mom T. Unstable distortion-product otoacoustic emission phase in Meniere's disease. *Hear Res* 2011;277(1-2) :88-95.

[29] de Kleine E, Mateijsen DJM, Wit HP, Albers FWJ. Evoked otoacoustic emissions in patients with Ménière's disease. *Otol Neurotol* 2002;23(4):510-516.

[30] Eggermont JJ, Schmidt PH. Meniere's disease: a long-term follow-up study of hearing loss. *Ann Otol Rhinol Laryngol* 1985;94:1-9.

[31] Brown DJ, Gibson WP. On the differential diagnosis of Ménière's disease using low-frequency acoustic biasing of the 2f1-f2 DPOAE. *Hear Res* 2011;282(1-2):119-127.

[32] Martin GK, Ohlms LA, Franklin DJ, Harris FP, Lonsbury-Martin BL. Distortion Product Emission in Humans: Influence of sensorineural hearing loss. *Ann Otol Rhinol Laryngol* 1990;99(suppl):30-42.

[33] Dauman R, Aran JM, Portmann M. Summating potential and water balance in Meniere's disease. *Ann Otol Rhinol Laryngol* 1986;95:389-395

[34] Buki B, Avan P, Lemaire JJ, Dordain M, Chazal J, Ribari O. Otoacoustic emissions: a new tool for monitoring intracranial pressure changes through stapes displacements. *Hear Res* 1996;94(1-2):125-139

[35] Rotter A, Weikert S, Hensel J, Scholz G, Scherer H, Holzl M. Low-frequency distortion product otoacoustic emission test compared to ECoG in diagnosing endolymphatic hydrops. *Eur Arch Otorhinolaryngol* 2008;265(6):643-649.

[36] van Huffelen WM, Mateijsen NJ, Wit HP. Classification of patients with Meniere's disease using otoacoustic emissions. *Audiol Neurotol* 1998;3(6):419-430.

[37] Hall JW III. Handbook of Otoacoustic Emissions, Singular Thomson learning. 2000; pp. 517-521.

[38] Nubel K, Kabudwand E, Scholz G, Mrowinski D. Diagnosis of endolymphatic hydrops with low tone masked otoacoustic emissions. *Laryngorhinootologie* 1995;74(11):651-656

[39] Hof-Duin NJ, Wit HP. Evaluation of low-frequency biasing as a diagnostic tool in Meniere patients. *Hear Res* 2007;231(1-2):84-89.

[40] Hatzopoulos S, Cheng J, Grzanka A, Martini A. Time-frequency analyses of TEOAE recordings from normal and SNHL patients. *Audiology* 2000;39(1):1-12

[41] Mom T, Montalban A, Bascoul A, Gilain L, Avan P. Acoustic phase shift: objective evidence for intra-labyrinthine pressure disturbance in Meniere's disease provided by otoacoustic emissions. *Eur Ann Otorhinoralyngol Head Neck Dis* 2012;129(1):17-21.

[42] Büki B, Avan P, Lemaire JJ, Dordain M, Chazal J, Ribari O. Otoacoustic emissions: a new tool for monitoring intracranial pressure changes through stapes displacements. *Hear Res* 1996;94 (4):125-139

[43] Avan P, Lemaire JJ, Drdain M, Chazal J, Buki B, Ribari O. Otoacoustic emissions and monitoring of intracranial hypertension. *J Audiol Med* 1998; 7(1):46-57.

[44] Inoue Y, Kanzaki J, O-Ushi T, Ogawa K, Ogata A, Yoshihara S, Satoh Y. Clinical application of transiently evoked otoacoustic emissions after glycerol administration for diagnosis of sensorineural hearing loss. *Ausis Nasus Larynx* 1997;24:143-149.

[45] Sakashita T, Kubo T, Kyunai K, Ueno K, Hikawa C, Shibata T, Yamane H, Kusuki M, Wada T, Uyama T. Changes in otoacoustic emissions during the glycerol test in the ears of patients with Meniere's disease. *Nihon Jibiinkoka Gakkai Kaiho* 2001;104(6):682-693.

Section 6

Ménière's Disease and Tinnitus

Chapter 11

Ménière's Disease and Tinnitus

Ricardo Rodrigues Figueiredo,

Andréia Aparecida de Azevedo and

Norma de Oliveira Penido

Additional information is available at the end of the chapter

http://dx.doi.org/10.5772/66390

Abstract

Tinnitus is one of the Ménière's disease clue symptoms, but by far less studied than vertigo or other types of dizziness. The typical Ménière's tinnitus is a low pitched fluctuating one. Although controversial, cochlear Ménière's disease may account for a tinnitus subtype, a fact that may impact on tinnitus diagnosis and treatment. Further studies focused on tinnitus are necessary to clarify at which extent Ménière's disease may have a role in some types of chronic tinnitus.

Keywords: tinnitus, Ménière's disease, hearing loss, vertigo, dizziness

1. Introduction

Ménière disease (MD) is a chronic inner ear condition that was first described by Prosper Ménière in the nineteenth century [1]. His initial description of the disease including hearing loss, vertigo and tinnitus was accurate, but the pathophysiology of the condition was only described 75 years later. The endolymphatic hydrops is the main finding, initially ascertained only in post-mortem exams and nowadays detectable in high resolution magnetic resonance imaging (MRI) [2].

The reported prevalence of MD is 190–513/100,000 cases [3]. Classical symptoms include fluctuating hearing loss, aural fullness and periodic vertigo and tinnitus [2]. The diagnosis criteria from the American Academy of Otolaryngology and Head and Neck Surgery (AAO-HNS)

INTECH
open science | open minds

© 2017 The Author(s). Licensee InTech. This chapter is distributed under the terms of the Creative Commons Attribution License (http://creativecommons.org/licenses/by/3.0), which permits unrestricted use, distribution, and reproduction in any medium, provided the original work is properly cited.

and the Bárány Society do not recognize an eventual 'cochlear' Ménière disease [4], but recent imaging studies (gadolinium contrasted 3T MRI) are more sympathetic with this possibility [5].

Although virtually all patients that fulfilled the AAO-HNF clinical criteria for MD whose inner ears were evaluated post-mortem exhibited endolymphatic hydrops (EH), not all the patients with Proven EH developed MD [2]. Many theories concerning the pathophysiology of MD have been proposed, including changes in endolymph reabsorption due to anatomical variations, perfusion/reperfusion vascular changes, autoimmune mechanisms and changes in water homeostasis [6]. Aquaporins (AQP) are involved in fluid regulation in the inner ear, specifically the subtypes AQP 1, 4 and 6 [6, 7]. It has been demonstrated that vasopressin and oxytocin have a direct effect on aquaporin-mediated regulation of inner ear fluids [7]. Moreover, cytochemical changes in AQP 4 and 6 expressions in the cochlear supporting cells were demonstrated in MD inner ears [6].

2. Current trends of thoughts concerning tinnitus pathophysiology

Tinnitus is the perception of noise which is not generated by external stimulus [8]. It affects approximately 25% of the general population; one third on a frequent basis [9]. Tinnitus may be classified as auditory and para-auditory tinnitus, with the former representing the majority of cases and the latter being subdivided into muscular and vascular tinnitus, sometimes referred as somatosounds [10].

According to the most recent trends of thought, tinnitus is not considered a disease, but a symptom, which may have multiple causes, sometimes even in a single patient [11, 12]. Noise exposure, metabolic and cardiovascular disease, presbycusis, ototoxicity and cranial and cervical trauma are the most frequently considered causes of tinnitus [12, 13]. Caffeine abuse, dietary factors, temporomandibular joint and cervical diseases have also been described as contributing factors [14–16].

Tinnitus is believed to be a central phenomenon that follows an initial peripheral damage [17–19]. The cochlear and/or auditory nerve damage may be permanent, temporary or even subclinical and central neuroplasticity, including decrease of efferent inhibition, tonotopical reorganization and activation of, or modulation by, non-auditory areas have been demonstrated to account for many tinnitus features [17, 18]. Despite the general consensus regarding the role of peripheral damage on the onset of tinnitus, many other factors contribute to tinnitus distress [20]. The correlation of tinnitus improvement and hearing loss recovery in sudden sensorineural hearing loss exists, but is not robust [20]. Nevertheless, peripheral aspects of tinnitus may not be ruled out even in chronic tinnitus, considering that around 45% of the patients submitted to VIII pair neurectomy experimented tinnitus improvement [21]. Ménière disease, particularly, may be an important example of 'peripheral' tinnitus, considering that in the initial stages tinnitus (as well as the other symptoms) is intermittent and acute, with no sufficient time for the arousal of a fully manifested neuroplasticity.

http://dx.doi.org/10.5772/66390

3. Tinnitus characteristics in Ménière disease

According to the criteria of AAO-HNS, MD clue symptoms are recurrent vertigo, fluctuating hearing loss and tinnitus or aural fullness sensation [4, 22]. Tinnitus is probably the less studied of these symptoms, although specific characteristics of MD tinnitus have been observed [23].

First of all, tinnitus is rarely one of the first symptoms noticed (vertigo is the usual one) [23]. Tinnitus is reported by 94% of the patients and considered important by 37% of them [24]. As the years pass and MD disease attacks become more frequent, tinnitus may become permanent and more severe [23, 24].

As tinnitus is usually related to hearing loss, it is not a surprise that MD tinnitus is often low frequencies tinnitus (125/250 Hz) [23]. Nevertheless, according to some studies, this low pitched tinnitus is better tolerated than the high pitched ones [23].

Tinnitus was found to be a less disabling symptom than vertigo by most of the patients [23]. Nevertheless, some patients consider tinnitus an important symptom, and for 19% of MD patients, tinnitus is the most severe complaint, although not associated with a relevant impact in general health and quality of life [24, 25]. According to some studies, the severity of tinnitus does not seem to correlate with the severity of vertigo attacks [23], suggesting that vestibular and cochlear aspects of MD may be independent at some level. On the other hand, some studies demonstrated a strong association between tinnitus and other Ménière symptoms [26].

Diuretics have been proposed as a valuable treatment for Ménière's disease, although the level of evidence concerning their efficacy is low [27]. The eventual side effects of diuretic therapy must not be ruled out as a co-factor for tinnitus development, if we consider it direct ototoxicity and the possibility of excessive decrease of the blood pressure, which, according to some authors, may account for direct perfusion/reperfusion changes in the inner ear [27].

The controversial issue concerning the hypothetical 'cochlear Ménière' is still a challenge. Current AAO-HNS definitions do not allow this possibility [22], but there is some evidence that it might exists [28–30], so it opens a window for the establishment of a tinnitus subtype. According to some authors, MD may begin with cochlear symptoms only, which may be attributed to other diseases related to hearing loss [30]. According to one study, tinnitus is the first symptom in 6.6% of the cases and the median time frame to develop the symptomatic triad in such cases is 3 years [30]. Having said so, it may be possible that cochlear symptoms occur without vertigo, at least for an initial time frame. The Ménière's Disease Index (MDI) was developed as an objective correlation of MD, based on audiometric (pure-tone audiometry air threshold at 125 Hz and pure-tone audiometry air threshold at 8000 Hz) and transtympanic electrocochleography (summation potential amplitude at 4000 Hz) data [28]. A recent study evaluated the MDI scores in patients with audiological symptoms and without vertigo, concluding that the 'cochlear MD' patients may represent a separate clinical entity, with MD's resembling pathophysiology and/or endolymphatic hydrops ('Ménière-like') [29]. A typical case is represented below. **Figure 1** shows the audiometric findings of a possible cochlear Ménière disease with tinnitus. This is a 32-year-old woman with complaints of tinnitus and aural fullness at the right ear. She had no vertigo or

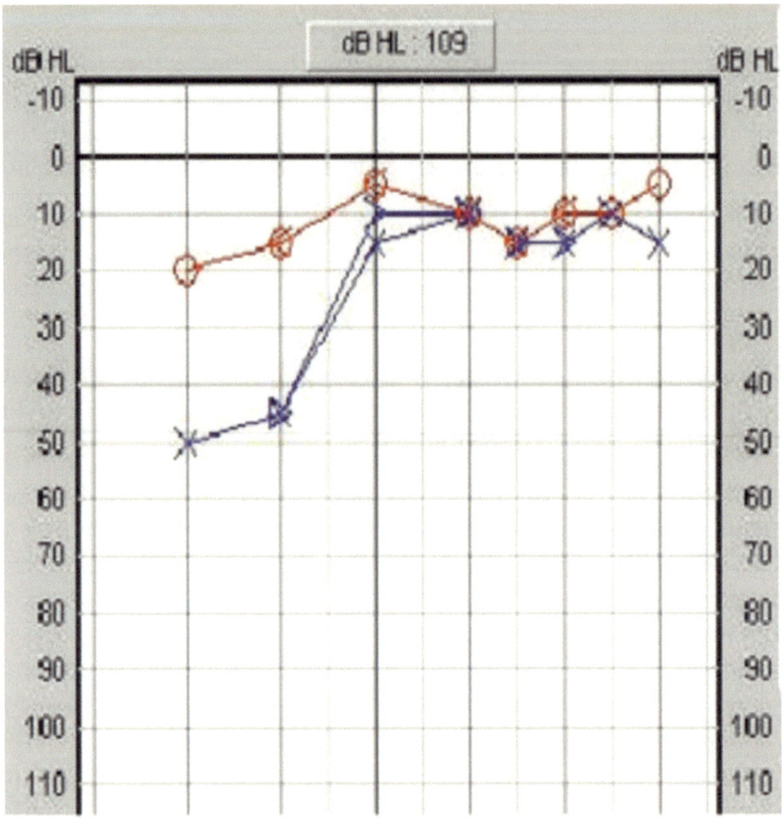

Figure 1. Pure tone audiometry of a 32-year-old woman with left year tinnitus pitched at 250 Hz and no vertigo or other forms of dizziness/imbalance. Intracanal ECoG showed a high SP/AP ratio (40%) in the left ear. This may represent a cochlear form of MD with tinnitus as the sole complaint.

other forms of dizziness or imbalance. Physical otolaryngological exam was normal. Pure tone audiometry revealed a mild sensorineural hearing loss at the low frequencies on the right ear. Tinnitus pitch matching was centred in 250 Hz. The electrocochleography with ear canal electrode showed a high SP/AP relationship (40%) in the right ear. This may represent a typical case of 'cochlear Ménière' in which tinnitus was the major complaint.

4. Possible treatment implications

Tinnitus treatment is still a challenge. There is no FDA-approved drug for tinnitus treatment and most of the clinical trials with drugs were not replicated, probably due to differences in the samples, tinnitus characteristics, methodology and drug dosage [31]. According to the recent consensus of the AAO-HNS, treatment should focus on counselling, auditory stimulation and cognitive behavioural therapy [11]. On the other hand, according to many researchers there is no reason that tinnitus could not be pharmacologically targeted, considering the multiple neurotransmitters and receptors involved in tinnitus pathophysiology [32]. The main goal of pharmacological treatment is to deliver the drug, to the right place, in the right amount, in other words, subtyping tinnitus. Understanding the neurochemistry at the peripheral and central areas involved in tinnitus is an important path to follow and may result in the development of successful therapies [31]. Following this line of thinking, if there should be a Ménière's related tinnitus, this could be a possible pharmacological target.

There is a general lack of studies that analyse the effects of MD treatment on tinnitus distress. In a retrospective study comparing patients with vestibular disorders that were treated or not with betahistine 24 mg bid, tinnitus improvement was significantly better in the group treated with betahistine [33]. There was no mention of the type of vestibular disorders included. These findings, although not specific for MD, may encourage further studies, considering that higher doses of betahistine (even reaching 288–480 mg/day) that have been safely employed to MD treatment could also be tried at patients with tinnitus [34].

Recently, it has been demonstrated that nasal oxytocin could induce an immediate decrease in tinnitus volume [35]. Oxytocin and vasopressin receptors are found at the cochlea and were demonstrated to be related to fluid regulation in the inner ear, via inner ear AQPs [6]. Although central effects of oxytocin may also play a role in tinnitus treatment, this immediate effect may be related to some kind of hydrops reduction.

In the last years, cochlear implants have been indicated for alleviating tinnitus, with encouraging results [11]. One study evaluated the effects of cochlear implants in patients with severe sensorineural hearing loss and Ménière's disease. Tinnitus distress, evaluated by the Tinnitus Handicap Inventory (THI) questionnaire, was significantly reduced in patients with MD (14 points decrease 6 months after the implantation, $p = 0.002$) [36].

5. Conclusions

Although, tinnitus is well known as a component of MD spectrum of symptoms, there is some evidence that it may occur alongside with other auditory symptoms in the absence of vertigo or other forms of dizziness. Understanding MD as a possible tinnitus subtype may unveil an important opportunity to study further tinnitus treatment strategies, such as betahistine, oxytocin and cochlear implants.

Author details

Ricardo Rodrigues Figueiredo[1,2]*, Andréia Aparecida de Azevedo[2,3] and Norma de Oliveira Penido[3]

*Address all correspondence to: rfigueiredo@otosul.com.br

1 Faculdade de Medicina de Valença, Valença, RJ, Brazil

2 Tinnitus Research Initiative Pharmagroup

3 Universidade Federal de São Paulo, SP, Brazil

References

[1] Atkinson M. Ménière's original papers reprinted with an English translation with commentaries and biographical sketch. Acta Otolaryngolica. 1961;**162**:1-78

[2] Gürkov R, Pyyko I, Kentala F. What is Ménière's disease? A contemporary re-evaluation of endolymphatic hydrops. Journal of Neurology. 2016;**263**(1):71-81. DOI: 10.1007/s00415-015-7930-1

[3] Havia M, Kentala E, Pyykö I. Prevalence of MD in general population of Southern Finland. Otolaryngology Head and Neck Surgery. 2005;**133**(5):762-768

[4] Lopez-Escamez JA, Carey J, Chung W, Goebel JA, Magnusson M, Mandala M et al. Diagnostic criteria for Menière's disease. Journal of Vestibular Research. 2015;**25**:1-7. DOI: 10.3233/VES-150549

[5] Pyykö I, Nakashima T, Yoshida T, Zou J, Naganawa S. Ménière's disease: A reappraisal supported by a variable latency of symptoms and the MRI visualization of endolymphatic hydrops. British Medical Journal Open. 2013;**3**(2). DOI: 10.1136/bmjopen-2012-001555

[6] Ishiyama G, Lopez IA, Sepahdari AR, Ishiyama A. Meniere's disease: Histopatology, cytochemistry and imaging. Annals of the NewYork Academy of Sciences. 2015;**22**:1-9. DOI: 10.1111/nyas.12699

[7] Eckhard A, Gleiser C, Arnold H, Rask-Andersen H, Kumagami H, Müller M et al. Water channel proteins in the inner ear and their link to hearing impairment and deafness. Molecular Aspects of Medicine. 2012;**33**(5-6):612-37. DOI: 10.1016/j.mam.2012.06.004

[8] Heller AJ. Classification and epidemiology of tinnitus. Otolaryngologic Clinics of North America. 2003;**36**(2):239-248

[9] Shargorodsky J, Curhan GC, Farwell WR. Prevalence and characteristics of tinnitus among US adults. The American Journal of Medicine. 2010;**123**(8):711-718. DOI: 10.1016/j.amjmed.2010.02.015

[10] Herraiz C, Aparicio JM. Diagnostic clues in pulsatile tinnitus (somatosounds). Acta Otorrinolaringológica Española. 2007;**58**(9):426-433

[11] Langguth B, Kreuzer PM, Kleinjung T, De Ridder D. Tinnitus: Causes and clinical management. The Lancet Neurology. 2013;**12**(9):920-930. DOI: 10.1016/S1474-4422(13)70160-1

[12] Tunkel DE, Bauer CA, Sun GH, Rosenfeld RM, Chandrasekhar SS, Cunningham ER Jr et al. Clinical practice guideline: Tinnitus. Journal of Otolaryngology Head and Neck Surgery. 2014;**151**(2):1-40. DOI: 10.1177/0194599814545325

[13] Henry JA, Dennis KC, Schechter MA. General review of tinnitus: prevalence, mechanisms, effects and management. Journal of Speech Language and Hearing Research. 2005;**48**(5):49-70

[14] Rocha CB, Sanchez TG. Efficacy of myofascial trigger point deactivation for tinnitus control. Brazilian Journal of Otorhinolaryngology. 2012;**78**(6):21-26

[15] Ferendiuk E, Zajdel K, Pihut M. Incidence of otolaryngological symptoms in patients with temporomandibular joint dysfunctions. BioMed Research International. 2014;**2014**:824684.DOI:10.1155/2014/824684.Epub 2014 Jun 24.

[16] Figueiredo RR, Rates MJ, Azevedo AA, Moreira RK, Penido NO. Effects of the reduction of caffeine consumption on tinnitus perception. Brazilian Journal of Otorhinolaryngology. 2014;**80**(5):416-421. DOI: 10.1016/j.bjorl.2014.05.033

[17] Møller A. The role of auditory deprivation. In: Møller A, Langguth B, DeRidder D, Kleinjung T, editors. Textbook of Tinnitus. New York: Springer; 2011. pp 95-98. DOI: 10.1007/978-1-60761-145-5

[18] Møller A. The role of neural plasticity in tinnitus. In: Møller A, Langguth B, DeRidder D, Kleinjung T, editors. Textbook of Tinnitus. New York: Springer; 2011.pp. 99-102. DOI: 10.1007/978-1-60761-145-5

[19] Eggermont JJ. The Neural Synchrony Model of Tinnitus. In: Eggermont JJ,editor. The Neuroscience of Tinnitus. Oxford: Oxford University Press; 2012.pp. 154-173

[20] Nogueira-Neto FB, Gallardo FP, Suzuki FA, Penido NdeO. Prognostic and evolutive factors of tinnitus triggered by sudden sensorineural hearing loss. Otology & Neurotology. 2016;**37**(6):627-633. DOI: 10.1097/MAO.0000000000001049

[21] House JW, Brackmann DE. Tinnitus: Surgical treatment. Ciba Foundation Symposium. 1981;**85**:204-216

[22] Committee on Hearing and Equilibrium guidelines for the diagnosis and evaluation of therapy in Ménière's Disease. American Academy of Otolaryngology – Head and Neck Foundation Inc. Otolaryngology Head Neck Surgery. 1995;**113**:181-185

[23] Sánchez IR, Garrigues HP, Rivera VR. Clinical characteristics of tinnitus in Ménière's disease. Acta Otorrinolaringológica Española. 2010;**61**(5):327-331.DOI: 10.1016/j.otorrino.2010.06.004

[24] Yoshida T, Stephens D, Kentala E, Levo H, Auramo Y, Poe D et al. Tinnitus complaint behaviour in long-standing Ménière's disorder:its association with other cardinal symptoms. Clinical Otolaryngology. 2011;**36**:461-467. DOI: 10.111/j.1749-4486.2011.02381.x

[25] Stephens D, Pyykkö I, Yoshida T, Kentala E, Levo H, Auramo Y et al. The consequences of tinnitus in long-standing Ménière's disease. Auris Nasus Larynx 2012;**39**:469-474. DOI: 10-1016/j.anl.2011.10.011

[26] Yardley L, Dibb B, Osborne G. Factors associated with quality of life in Ménière's disease. Clinical Otolaryngology and Allied Sciences. 2003;**28**:436-441

[27] Pirodda A, Ferri GG, Raimondi MC, Borghi C. Diuretics in Meniere disease: A therapy or a potential cause of harm? Medical Hypotheses. 2011;**77**:869-871. DOI: 10.1016/j.medy.2011.07.060

[28] Claes GM, De Valck CFJ, Van de Heyning PH, Wuyts FL. The Ménière's Disease Index: An objective correlate of Ménière's disease, based on audiometric and electrocochleographic data. Otology and Neurotology. 2011;**32**:887-892. DOI: 10.1097/MAO.0b013e318219ff9a

[29] Claes GM, De Valck CFJ, Van de Heyning P, Wuyts FL. Does 'Cochlear Ménière's Disease' exist? An electrocochleographic and audiometric study. Audiology and Neurotology. 2013;**18**:63-70. DOI: 10.1159/000342686

[30] Belinchon A, Perez-Garrigues H, Tenias JM. Evolution of symptoms in Ménière's disease. Audiology Neurotology. 2012;**17**:126-132. DOI: 10.1159/000331945

[31] Figueiredo RR, Azevedo AA, Penido NO. Pharmacological treatment of tinnitus. In. Watson J,editor. Tinnitus Epidemiology, Causes and Emerging Therapeutic Treatments. New York: Nova Science Publishers; 2016.pp 25-42

[32] Langguth B, Salvi R, Elgoyhen AB. Emerging pharmacotherapy of tinnitus. Expert Opinion and Emerging Drugs. 2009;**14**(4):687-702. DOI: 10.1517/14728210903206975

[33] Ganança MM, Caovilla HH, Gazzola JM, Ganança CF, Ganança FF. Betahistine in the treatment of tinnitus in patients with vestibular disorders. Brazilian journal of otorhinolaryngology. 2011;**77**(4):499-503

[34] Lezius F, Adrion C, Mansmann U, Jahn K, Strupp M. High dosage betahistine dihydrochloride between 288 and 480 mg/day in patients with severe Ménière's disease: A case series. European Archives of Otorhinolaryngology. 2011;**268**(8):1237-1240.DOI: 10.1007/s00405-011-1647-2

[35] Azevedo, A, Figueiredo RR, Schlee W. Immediate effects of nasal oxytocin in tinnitus patients. In: Annals of the 10th International Tinnitus Research Initiative Conference; 16-18 March 2016; Nottingham, England. Nottingham: Tinnitus Research Initiative; 2016.pp 61-62

[36] Mick P, Amoodi H, Arnoldner C, Shipp D, Friesen L, Lin V et al. Cochlear implantation in patients with advanced Ménière's disease. Otology Neurotology. 2014;**35**(7):1172-1178. DOI: 10.1097/MAO0000000000000202

Section 7

Ménière's Disease Treatment

Chapter 12

Meniere's Disease Treatment

Eduardo Amaro Bogaz,
André Freitas Cavallini da Silva,
Davi Knoll Ribeiro and Gabriel dos Santos Freitas

Additional information is available at the end of the chapter

http://dx.doi.org/10.5772/67981

Abstract

The Meniere's disease is a chronic condition that requires treatment for long time and whose control is not always easy to achieve, requiring some multidrug treatments, and sometimes even procedures. We have many drugs and procedures to the treatment of Meniere's disease which may be taken according to the stage of disease and individual features.

Keywords: Meniere's disease, treatment, endolymphatic hypertension, betahistine, diuretics, endolymphatic surgery

1. Introduction

Meniere's disease (MD) symptoms are caused by the accumulation of endolymph in the membranous labyrinth, with consequent endolymphatic hypertension, that has been demonstrated in anatomical-pathological studies [1]. Endolymphatic hypertension leads to malfunction or irreversible damage to the sensory cells of the anterior and posterior labyrinths with their consequent symptoms. It is a multifactorial disorder and involves the participation of genetic and external factors.

The treatment of Meniere's symptoms is based on the control and reversal of endolymphatic hypertension which can be done through medications, change in life habits, and others. Conservative treatments are aimed at normalizing the membranous labyrinth system homeostasis and controlling the evolution of the disease as well as its symptoms. When symptom control cannot be achieved by conservative treatments, one can consider using invasive treatments that may assist in the control of endolymphatic hypertension, or destroy the labyrinth sensory cells.

INTECH
open science | open minds

© 2017 The Author(s). Licensee InTech. This chapter is distributed under the terms of the Creative Commons Attribution License (http://creativecommons.org/licenses/by/3.0), which permits unrestricted use, distribution, and reproduction in any medium, provided the original work is properly cited.

It is worth noting that the clinical spectrum of Meniere's disease is broad, with the possibility of remission and recurrence of symptoms, and even very unfavorable evolution, with irreversible hearing loss and permanent damage to the vestibular function. A good treatment must be individualized for each patient, taking into consideration such possibilities, the stage of the disease, and the possible consequences that have been promoted.

The more common treatments include salt restriction, diuretics and betahistine, intratympanic gentamicin and steroids, ablative surgical therapies and endolymphatic sac surgery, and Meniett device. Many ways of hearing and vestibular rehabilitation are available for chronic damage treatment, according to each situation (**Table 1**).

Treatment	Level of evidence
Salt restriction	5
Diuretics	2b
Betahistine	2b
Steroids	1b
Gentamicin	1b
Endolymphatic sac surgery	2b
Vestibular nerve section	2b
Labyrinthectomy	2b
Meniett device	No evidence level

Table 1. Level of evidence of treatments according to the Oxford Centre for evidence-based medicine.

2. Treatment modalities

2.1. Salt restriction and other dietary modifications

The observation that water retention can exacerbate the symptoms of Meniere's disease (MD) was first documented in 1929 [2]. Studies on the increase of sodium levels inducing hydrops attacks have been performed since then, with numerous related publications [3]. More recent studies also suggest that the restriction of salt, associated with the use of diuretics, gets better symptom control in patients with Meniere's disease [4]. The endolymph disturbances of volume and electrolytes are the main cause of the symptoms experienced by patients with MD. High salt intake can affect the concentration of electrolytes in the blood, which affects the composition of endolymph. This fluctuation in the composition and volume of endolymph contributes to the floating nature of symptoms experienced by people suffering from MD [5].

A low-salt diet is an important treatment for patients with MD. The effectiveness of treatment is shown when sodium intake is reduced to less than 3 g per day. A low-salt diet can induce an increase in plasma concentration of aldosterone, which can enable the transport of ions to the absorption of endolymph in the endolymphatic sac. Other dietary changes include limiting alcohol and caffeine intake as evidenced by [4]. Both alcohol and caffeine can lead to vasoconstriction and a decrease in blood supply to the inner ear which can make the symptoms of patients more intense.

2.2. Diuretics in Meniere's symptoms

Diuretics affect the balance of electrolytes in the endolymph, leading to the reduction of the volume and pressure, which can occur by increased drainage of endolymph or by reducing its production. They are usually used to control vertigo, hearing loss, tinnitus, and aural fullness in patients with Meniere's disease.

The article published by Ref. [6] makes an analysis of the retrospective medical records of patients with Meniere's disease and was designed to evaluate the effect of acetazolamide and chlorthalidone at the rate of hearing loss. Three groups were compared as follows: (1) 79 patients treated with clortalidona from 5 to 13.4 years; (2) 42 patients treated with acetazolamide between 5 and 7.8 years; and (3) a control group of 71 patients who received only the symptomatic treatment for intermittent dizziness, followed by 5–24.1 years. In the short-term, after 2–6 weeks of treatment, a statistically significant reduction of average hearing loss was observed with both clorotalidona and acetazolamide. In the long run, more than 5 years, no preventive effect on the deterioration of hearing loss can be detected. Both acetazolamide and chlorthalidone may be useful for diagnostic purposes, causing a fluctuation of hearing, as well as to control the attacks of vertigo, but is not useful for the long-term prevention of deterioration in hearing on Meniere's disease [6].

Another double-blind randomized controlled study published in 1982 [7] comparing the betahistine use with hydrochlorothiazide. Patients were initially kept under observation for 3 months without medication beyond symptomatics. Then patients were divided into two groups, each with 16 patients receiving betahistine or hydrochlorothiazide during 6 months. Before and during treatment, subjective symptoms, such as dizziness, bouts of dizziness, tinnitus, aural fullness, and general well-being, were evaluated every 4 weeks. At the moment, betahistine seems to be the drug of choice for Meniere's disease with floating hearing thresholds. In all patients of this study, an improvement and reduction in the severity, frequency, and duration of vertigo attacks in 6 months of treatment was observed. In contrast, hydrochlorothiazide showed a distinct therapeutic effect on general well-being and vertigo, notably during the first months of treatment in patients with stable hearing thresholds [7].

Klockhoff et al. in 1976 [8] observed 34 patients with Meniere's disease who were treated with chlorthalidone. Twenty-six patients had drug-related improvements, especially a reduction in the prevalence and severity of vertigo. In four patients, the effect was minor, other four patients seemed to have resistance to chlorthalidone despite positive glycerin tests, and two of them needed surgery. Chlorthalidone was also given to 220 severely disabled patients who were hospitalized for further examination and possible surgical procedure. The improvements were obtained in such a way that the operation was avoided in 133 patients (60%).

Regular or long-term treatment with chlorthalidone that produces a symptomatic relief is considerable in many patients during the active phase of the disease. It reduces the need for surgical intervention and helps patients to maintain an active life, but not arrest the course of degenerative disease [8].

However, Brookes and Booth [9] published an observational study that was conducted in 14 patients who received acetazolamide with duration ranging from 1 week to 9 months and the therapeutic efficacy of this medication. There was improvement in four patients and improvement was not maintained in two of these, while the other had to cease the medication due to the development of kidney stone. The worsening of symptoms was observed in 3 cases and adverse side effects were observed in 6 of the 13 patients (46.2%) that fulfilled the dosage of drugs. It is suggested that this high incidence of side effects can be consistent with the general metabolic difference between Meniere's disease patients and normal individuals. This work concluded that acetazolamide has no place in the medical treatment of Meniere's disease [9].

More recently, a new review conducted by Duke University in 2016, based on boots with diuretics in MD for the last 10 years sought to assess, including any oral diuretic study in adult patients, hearing results reported, results of vestibular symptoms, effects, and complications of diuretic treatment. In this revision, 19 studies were included with considerable heterogeneity in the population of patients evaluated, design of studies, as well as type of diuretics, dosage, follow-up, and results. Most of these studies reported improvement in vestibular symptoms, but little improvement of hearing in these patients. As with other conditions faced by otorhinolaryngologists, diuretic therapy for Meniere's disease is often initiated as first-line therapy, although low level of evidence is present to justify its use (2b) [10].

Last survey of Cochrane [11] found no evidence of high quality to evaluate the efficacy of diuretics on Meniere's disease to not to introduce controlled double-blind randomized trials using placebo for diagnosis and outcome evaluation. Despite the lack of evidence of high quality, some studies have reported an improvement in patients' vertigo during use of diuretics in the short-term.

2.3. Betahistine on Meniere's symptoms

Betahistine is a drug that has pharmacological and structural properties similar to histamine. Betahistine is a heteroreceptor H3 antagonist and agonist H1 receiver that improves the microcirculation in the inner ear, promoting and facilitating central vestibular compensation [12]. The circulatory effects of betahistine have been demonstrated in laboratory animals and in humans. Betahistine increases the regional blood flow in patients with degenerative cerebrovascular disease and significantly improves cognitive function in the elderly [13].

Mira et al., in 2003 [14], compared the efficacy and safety of betahistine dihydrochloride to placebo in recurring dizziness resulting from Meniere's disease (MD) or benign paroxysmal positional vertigo (BPPV) of vascular origin. In this double-blind, parallel-group, multicenter, and randomized study, a group was treated with betahistine (MD: 34/BPPV: 41) and another with placebo (MD: 40/BPPV: 29). Betahistine had a significant effect on the intensity, frequency, and duration of vertigo's attacks compared with placebo, also with a better quality of life [14].

Lezius et al. [15] evaluated the clinical benefits and side effects of high doses of betahistine dihydrochloride (288–480 mg/day) in patients with severe Meniere's disease. In this series, 11 MD patients who have not responded well enough to 144 mg/day dosage of betahistina were treated individually with daily doses between 288 and 480 mg. As a result, the frequency and severity of dizziness were significantly reduced in all patients. The side effects were mild, Self-limited, and do not require any changes in treatment strategy. Despite the considerable limitations of an observational study, high doses of betahistine between 288 and 480 mg/day appear to be effective in patients who are not sufficient to respond to lower doses. In addition, these doses are well tolerated.

In contrast, Adrion et al. [16] indicate that the incidence of attacks related to Meniere's disease did not differ among the three treatment groups ($P = 0.759$). Compared with placebo, crisis rates were 1.036 (95% confidence interval −1.140 to 0.942) and 1.012 (0.919–1.114) to a betahistine low-dose and high-dose betahistine, respectively. The global monthly attack rate dropped significantly by 0.758 factor (0.705–0.816; $P < 0.001$). Based on the monthly average incidence population on average over the period of evaluation was of 2.722 (1.304–6.309), 3.204 (1.345–7.929), and 3.258 (1.685–7.266) for the placebo groups, betahistine low-dose and high-dose betahistine, respectively. The results were consistent with no important side effects. The placebo effect could not be evaluated.

The Cochrane survey [17] reveals no conclusion evidence of betahistine use on Meniere's treatment despite the good results.

2.4. H1 receptor blockers and calcium antagonist

H1 receptor blockers and calcium antagonist, flunarizine and cinnarizine, inhibit vasoconstriction and act as sedatives vestibular, being used in the treatment of central and peripheral vertigo. Both are contraindicated in patients with extrapyramidal disorders [13], being useful for symptomatic treatment and during crises.

2.5. Benzodiazepines

Benzodiazepines act in a way that increases the inhibitory effect of gamma-aminobutyric acid in the vestibular nuclei and is useful in the therapy of vertigo, in the control of anxiety, and panic attacks in patients dizzying. One may experience drowsiness, fatigue, and drug dependence.

2.6. The Ginkgo Biloba (EGb 761)

The EGb 761´s hemodynamic, hemorheological, metabolical, and neural effects are studied in Ref. [18]. It is used in the treatment of vertigo of peripheral origin [19].

Headache, hypotension, and gastrointestinal disturbance are the main adverse effects.

2.7. Intratympanic corticosteroid and Meniere's symptoms

The aim of these treatments is to use the medication that will affect the inner ear by entering the ear through the round window. Corticosteroids reduce the inflammation in the ear and can increase labyrinth circulation and also there have been some suggestions that the steroids affect the metabolism of salt in the inner ear [20].

In a retrospective analysis by She et al. [21] patients with intractable Meniere's disease were treated with intratympanic methylprednisolone perfusion. These 16 patients were followed for more than 2 years. The vertigo control rates in the short- and long-term were 94 and 81%, respectively; the improvements of functional activities in the short-term were 94 and 88% in the long-term. The tonal average did not change significantly. In patients with intractable disease with good hearing preservation, intratympanic methylprednisolone can control vertigo and functional improvement, being a viable alternative for an intractable Meniere's disease.

A retrospective analise performed by Boleas-Aguirre et al. states that control of dizziness was retrieved from 117 (91%) of 129 individuals and needed only 1 injection of dexamethasone 37%, 2 shots in 20%, 3 shots in 14%, and 4 injections in 8%; 21% needed more than 4 injections; 96 patients had follow-up data after 2 years. Of these, 91% had control of dizziness with intratympanic dexamethasone, and some needed more injections of dexamethasone or associated intratympanic gentamicin [22].

A review is published by the Cochrane in 2011 through randomized clinical trial of intratympanic dexamethasone versus placebo in patients with Meniere's disease. Only 22 patients were included. After 24 months of study, a statistically significant improvement in vertigo was confirmed compared to placebo. Change in score dizziness handicap inventory (60.4 against 41.3) and average improves subjective vertigo (90 versus 57%). The scheme of treatment described by the authors involves daily injections of dexamethasone 4 mg/ml solution for consecutive 5 days. These results were clinically significant. No complications were reported [23].

2.8. Intratympanic gentamicin injection

The first publication about the use of intratympanic aminoglycosides (streptomycin) on Meniere's disease in 1950 was of Schuknecht [24]. The aim of this therapy is to cause chemical damage or perform the ablation maze sick, in order to stop the floating labyrinth malfunction, causing the symptoms of Meniere's disease, and create a lasting situation of hypofunction where the brain can compensate for. This treatment can decrease the episodes of dizziness in Meniere's disease.

This chemical ablation of the labyrinth has some advantages over the classic surgical ablation (labyrinthectomy or vestibular nerve section), such as it can be performed on an outpatient basis under local anesthesia. Gentamicin is more vestibulotoxic than ototoxic, so it may be possible to preserve hearing. There is no consensus on the best dosing schedule to minimize hearing damage, but many authors argue that intermittent dosing with long intervals between two injections to check if hearing loss occurred is a safer approach in the maintenance of hearing [25].

The procedure is started after anesthesia of tympanic membrane topically with any phenol or EMLA® cream (2.5% lidocaine and 2.5% prilocaine). A small ventilation hole is made with a 25 gauge needle preferably earlier, and then the drug is injected postinferiorly until the middle ear space bottom is filled. The patient is then instructed to keep the ear where it was

http://dx.doi.org/10.5772/67981

injected the drug up to 20 min, to allow for absorption by the round window. In most studies, the application of gentamicin dose varies from 30 to 40 mg/mL (1 vial), applied between 6 weeks and 6 months, or 12 shots with a maximum of 360 mg, the following suggested ranges around 6–28 months, the American Academy of Otolaryngology Head and Neck Surgery (AAO-HNS) recommends a 2-year follow-up [26, 27].

Contraindications include active, middle ear infection only with hearing or ear balance function. The most commonly seen complications are hearing loss and unilateral vestibular hypofunction. Most of the patients need only an injection and most of these patients are able to avoid the ablative surgery due to significant improvement of treatment with intratympanic gentamicin.

The side effects of either intratympanic gentamicin or corticosteroids are minimal and a good result is achieved in about 90% with steroids at an early stage or gentamicin at a later stage, a very significant number when compared to the 30% success rate from placebo [28].

2.9. Endolymphatic sac surgery

Endolymphatic mastoid sac surgery (EMSS) has been known since the age of the Renaissance and remains a conservative popular procedure for the treatment of MD up to date [29]. Historically, vestibular neurectomy and transmastoid labyrinthectomy were provided to vestibular control, 90–95% of control rate. Vestibular neurectomy has a high potential for morbidity and neurosurgical complications. Hearing is eliminated in all cases of labyrinthectomy.

It is due to these possibilities of complications that today we opt for less destructive procedures to relieve vertigo.

In particular, EMSS appears to have regained popularity recently due to its low-risk safety profile, effectiveness in controlling episodes of vertigo, and in some cases improvement in hearing [30].

The procedure is initiated with the patient on general anesthesia and monitoring of the facial nerve. Antibiotics are administered and a standard mastoidectomy is performed followed by decompression of sigmoid sinus. Then the endolymphatic sac is identified behind the posterior semicircular canal, along the plate posterior fossa, below the Donaldson line. In a decompression surgery, bone about the sac is largely removed. A "stent" (Silastic® or Teflon®) is placed inside the sac that directs endolinfa to mastoid cavity or to the cerebrospinal fluid compartment. The more common contraindications are active mastoid or middle ear disease. Among complications related to this surgical procedure mainly are hearing loss, dizziness, cerebrospinal fluid loss, damage to the sigmoid sinus, facial palsy, addition of anesthetics, and general surgical risks. Within the surgical technique terms, similar results are achieved with decompression of the endolymphatic sac against shunting maneuvers.

Samy et al. concluded in a retrospective chart review of 456 consecutive patients between 1997 and 2006, that EMSS did not significantly affect hearing outcomes at 2-year follow-up. Of all patients in the study, 60% had no clinically significant change in hearing, whereas 24% improved and 16% worsened. The distribution of posttreatment hearing changes between the medical and surgical groups was statistically insignificant ($P = 17$) [31].

The safety of EMSS surgery has also been established in elderly patients with Meniere's disease. In a Paparella et al. study with 62 patients (age ≥ 65 years) submitted to 78 EMSS surgeries without significant complications, 1.6% of major complications, mainly cardiac arrhythmia and 77% of patients achieved complete resolution of the symptoms for up to 2 years after the procedure.

2.10. Vestibular nerve section (VNS)

The great brain surgeon Walther Edward Dandy (1886–1946) of Baltimore described the vestibular nerve section (VNS) in 1928. Until 1941, he had already operated 401 cases with only one fatality [31]. There was renewed interest in vestibular nerve section after House introduced the middle-fossa vestibular neurectomy in 1961. Fisch and Glasscock and colleagues modified House's middle-fossa approach to include inferior vestibular neurectomy for improved control of vertigo. Silverstein and Norrell described the first retrolabyrinthine vestibular nerve section for Meniere's disease [32].

Patients with bilateral vestibular disease are not considered for a VNS because of the oscillopsia and permanent imbalance that can result from bilateral vestibular loss.

Vestibular nerve section can be performed through a retrosigmoid approach or retrolabirintic, associated with the monitoring of the facial nerve and auditory evoked potential. In the retrosigmóide approach, lower and upper vestibular nerves are identified and divided in internal acoustic pores not taking care to injure the facial nerve or cochlear. The identification of the vestibular nerves can be facilitated by the decompression internal auditory canal laterally, in order to locate definitely references such as the horizontal and vertical ridges (Bill) and the unique nerve after semicircular canal ampulla.

Already in the retrolabirintic approach, a mastoidectomy is performed, with decompression of sigmoid sinus and posterior semicircular canal and the vertical segment of the facial nerve. The dura mater of the posterior fossa is then identified and the internal auditory meatus is decompressed to view individual nerves. The vestibular nerve and the facial cochlear are identified and the vestibular nerve is carefully cut with subsequent placement of fat graft inside the mastoidea cavity to prevent loss of CSF (cerebrospinal fluid). Central compensation after vestibular neurectomy is key for postoperative recovery of balance. This makes any indication of central nervous system diseases such as cerebellar dysfunction, multiple sclerosis, physiologic old age, and poor medical condition a relative contraindication for vestibular nerve section.

Vestibular nerve sectioning is one of the most effective procedures for treating intractable vertigo in patients with no hearing in a unilateral Meniere's disease ear. In the literature [33–37], vertigo control rates between 78 and over 90% have been reported.

The contraindications are rare for this type of surgery, complications can exemplify: loss of CSF, meningitis, cranial Neuropathies, seizures, stroke, and death, in addition to general surgical and anesthetic risks. One of the major setbacks of the postoperative period is the need for hospitalization of the patient around 2–5 days. Effective medical treatment and dietary control, combined with intermittent use of oral steroids and middle ear perfusion of steroids or gentamicin has substantially reduced the number of patients with intractable vertigo needing vestibular neurectomy.

2.11. Labyrinthectomy

The goal of the surgery is the removal of vestibular end organs of five neuroepithelium: the three semicircular canals, the utriculus, and sacculus. In patients with severe hearing loss who do not respond to other surgical and medical treatments, labyrinthectomy is typically the last choice for unilateral MD. Bilateral MD is a contraindication for this procedure, because of the oscillopsia and permanent imbalance that can result from bilateral vestibular loss, as for VNS.

Several studies have shown excellent control of vertigo in up to 97% of patients. There is a 3% risk of CSF leak and a 2% risk of facial nerve injury [38].

Classically indicated when the audiometry shows loss greater than 60 dB and discrimination less than 50%.

The patient is placed under general anesthesia and monitoring of facial nerve after antibiotic administration of a standard mastoidectomy is performed. The tegmen tympani, sigmoid sinus, horizontal channel, and facial nerves are all identified. Gain access to the horizontal semicircular canal, followed thereafter by posterior semicircular canal, which in turn is followed to the raw comunna to identify the upper channel of the semicircular canals to the lobby, and finally removes the sacculus and utriculus, after removal of all neuroepitélio, the surgical wound is closed and a bandage on the mastoid is applied.

It is normal to find the post or horizontal nystagmus and lateral superior oblique (LSO), a slope deviation can be occasionally observed due to acute interruption of the utricular unilateral entry. Complications include dizziness, loss of CSF, sigmoid sinus damage, facial paralysis, in addition to the anesthetic and surgical risks.

Often the vestibular therapy is useful in the postoperative period to assist the central compensation and the return to functionality.

Nevertheless, literature research concerning cases of labyrinthectomy and cochlear implantation in patients suffering Meniere's disease is limited and is being performed in cases of bilateral Meniere's disease or even 20 years after labyrinthectomy. Zwolan et al. performed to our knowledge the first simultaneous labyrinthectomy and cochlear implantation in a single patient [39]. As the results show, the combination of labyrinthectomy and cochlear implantation is an efficient concept for the treatment of patients with Meniere's disease and single-sided deafness in case where the above preconditions have been implemented. An excellent control of vertigo symptoms could be achieved using this therapeutical concept.

For patients with single-sided Meniere's disease and profound sensorineural hearing loss, a simultaneous labyrinthectomy and cochlear implantation are efficient method for the treatment of vertigo and rehabilitation of the auditory system [40].

3. Meniett device

During the decade of 1970, the demand for a more effective and a nondestructive method for the treatment of MD, Inglestad et al. [41] observed that some patients reported improvement with changes of pressure in a pressure chamber. Densert et al. [42] showed that the manipulation of the middle ear pressure influences the pressure in the inner ear; later, improved hearing and dizziness in patients with MD were described after the application of positive pressure in the middle ear.

Additionally, there was improvement of the cochlear electrical potentials after administration of positive pressure in the middle ear, which finally led to the development of the device known as the Meniett (Medtronic Xomed Surgical Products, Jacksonville, FL).

The Meniett device emits a pulse of repeated pressure of 0.6 second in the range of 0–20 cm H_2O at 6 Hz. Treatment consists of three to four cycles of a sequence of treatment of 5 min, this device requires only a short-term ventilation tube (Sheppard) to allow the transmission of impulses in an auditory external pressure to the middle ear.

The FDA approved the use of the device in 2002, demand is still low, despite recent work showing the effectiveness of the device. Meniett reduces the frequency of dizziness in patients with Meniere's disease activity, an improvement of AAO-HNS Meniere's disease functional level scale, but the device does not significantly improve hearing, showing a safe option for patients with refractory diseases to the conventional treatments [43].

4. Vestibular rehabilitation

Vestibular rehabilitation is a form of body and eye movement stimulation therapy designed to improve vestibular function and mechanisms of central adaptation and compensation. It is mainly useful to treat the MD squeal; vestibular adaptation exercises to prevent falls have proven to be particularly effective. This type of treatment is quite effective for patients with stabilized vestibular function [44].

5. Conclusion

Treatments in Meniere's disease are generally aimed at reducing the acute symptomology vertiginous episodes. The cure currently does not exist. To date, the treatment has convincingly been shown to be effective in altering the natural course of the disease, thereby preventing end organ damage, which results in hearing loss and vestibular impairment. The clinical spectrum of the disease of Meniere's symptoms is wide, with the possibility of remission and recurrence of symptoms, and even fairly unfavorable developments, with irreversible hearing loss and damage the vestibular function. A good treatment must be individualized for each patient, taking into consideration these possibilities, the stage of disease, and the possible consequences that have been promoted.

Author details

Eduardo Amaro Bogaz[1,2*], André Freitas Cavallini da Silva[1], Davi Knoll Ribeiro[1] and Gabriel dos Santos Freitas[1]

*Address all correspondence to: eabogaz@gmail.com

1 Department of Otolaryngology, São Camilo Hospital, São Paulo, Brazil

2 Department of Otology and Neurotology, São Camilo Hospital, São Paulo, Brazil

References

[1] Rauch SD, Merchant SN, Thedinger BA. Menière's syndrome and endolymphatic hydrops. Double-blind temporal bone study. Annals of Otology, Rhinology, and Laryngology. 1989;**98**:873-883

[2] Dederding D. Clinical and experimental examination in patients suffering from morbus Meniere including study of problems of bone conduction. Acta Oto-Laryngologica. 1929;**10**:1-156

[3] Furstenberg AC, Lashmet FH, Lathrop F. Meniere's symptom complex: medical treatment. Annals of Otology, Rhinology, and Laryngology. 1934;**43**:1035-1047

[4] Luxford E, Berliner KI, Lee J, Luxford, WM. Dietary modification as adjunct treatment in Méniere's disease: Patient willingness and ability to comply. Otology & Neurotology. 2013;**34**(8):1438-1443

[5] Hussain K, Murdin L, Schilder AGM. Restriction of salt intake and other dietary modifications for the treat-ment of Ménière's disease or syndrome. Cochrane Database of Systematic Reviews 2016, Issue 5. Art. No.: CD012173. DOI:10.1002/14651858.CD012 173. 1-9

[6] Corvera J, Corvera G. Long-term effect of acetazolamide and chlorthalidone on the hearing loss of Meniere's Disease. American Journal of Otology. 1989;**10**(2):142-145

[7] Petermann W, Mulch G. Long-term therapy of Meniere's disease. Comparison of effects of betahistine dihydrochloride and hydrochlorothiazide. Fortschritte der Medizin. 1982;**100**(10):431-435

[8] Klockhoff I, Lindblom U, Stahle J. Diuretic treatment of Meniere disease. Archives of Otolaryngology. 1974;**100**(4):262-265.

[9] Brookes GB, Booth JB. Oral acetazolamide in Meniere's disease. Journal of Laryngology and Otology. 1984;**98**(11):1087-1095

[10] Crowson MG, Patki A; Tucci DL. Uma revisão sistemática de diuréticos no tratamento médico de doença de Ménière. Otolaryngology – Head and Neck Surgery. 2016;**154**(5): 824-834

[11] Burgess A, Kundu S. Diuretics for Ménière's disease or syndrome. Cochrane Database of Systematic Reviews 2006, Issue 3. Art. No.: CD003599. DOI: 10.1002/14651858.CD003599.pub2. 1-14

[12] Lacour M, Sterkers O. Histamine and betahistine in the treatment of vertigo: Elucidation of mechanisms of action. CNS Drugs. 2001;**15**:853-870

[13] Van Cauwenberge PB, De Moor SE. Physiopathology of H3-receptors and pharmacology of betahistine. Acta Oto-laryngologica Supplementum. 1997;**526**:43-46

[14] Mira E, Guidetti G, Ghilardi L, Fattori B, Malannino N, Maiolino L, et al. Betahistine dihydrochloride in the treatment of peripheral vestibular vertigo. European Archives of Oto-Rhino-Laryngology. 2003;**260**(2):73-77

[15] Lezius F, Adrion C, Mansmann U, Jahn K, Strupp M. High-dosage betahistine dihydrochloride between 288 and 480 mg/day in patients with severe Meniere's disease: A case series. European Archives of Oto-rhino-laryngology. 2011;**268**:1237-1240

[16] Adrion C, et al. Efficacy and safety of betahistine treatment in patients with Meniere's disease: Primary results of a long term, multicentre, double blind, randomised, placebo controlled, dose defining trial (BEMED trial). British Medical Journal. 2016;**352**

[17] James A, Burton MJ. Betahistine for Ménière's disease or syndrome. Cochrane Database of Systematic Reviews 2001, Issue 1. Art. No.: CD001873. DOI: 10.1002/14651858.CD00 1873. 1-11

[18] Ganança MM, Munhoz MSL, Caovilla HH, Silva MLG. Managing vertigo. Hannover: Solvay; 2006/Clostre F. Ginkgo biloba extract (egb761): State of knowledge in the dawn of the year 2000. Annales Pharmaceutiques Francaises. 1999;**57**(Suppl 1):1S8-188.

[19] Ganança MM, Munhoz MSL, Caovilla HH, Silva, MLG. Managing vertigo. Hannover: Solvay; 2006/Cesarani A, Meloni F, Alpini D, Barozzi S, Verderio L, Boscani PF. Ginkgo biloba (egb 761) in the treatment of equilibrium disorders. Advances in Therapy. 1998;**15**(5):291-304

[20] Chi FL, Yang MQ, Zhou YD, Wang B. Therapeutic efficacy of topical application of dexamethasone to the round window niche after acoustic trauma caused by intensive impulse noise in guinea pigs. Journal of Laryngology and Otology. 2011;**125**(7):673-685

[21] She W, Lv L, Du X, Li H, Dai Y, Lu L, Ma X, Chen F. Long-term effects of intratympanic methylprednisolone perfusion treatment on intractable Ménière's disease. The Journal of Laryngology & Otology. 2015;**129**:232-237

[22] Boleas-Aguirre MS, Lin FR, Della Santina CC, Minor LB, Carey JP. Longitudinal results with intratympanic dexamethasone in the treatment of Ménière's disease. Otology & Neurotology. 2008;**29**(1):33-38

[23] Phillips JS, Westerberg B. Intratympanic steroids for Ménière's disease or syndrome. Cochrane Database of Systematic Reviews. 2011;**6**(7)

[24] Schuknecht HF. Ablation therapy for the relief of Meniere's disease. Laryngoscope. 1956;**66**:859-870

[25] Burneo JG, Montori VM, Faught E. Magnitude of the placebo effect in randomized trials of antiepileptic agents. Epilepsy & Behavior. 2002;**3**(6):532-534

[26] Postema RJ, Kingma, CM, Wit HP, Albers FW, Van Der Laan BF. Intratympanic gentamicin therapy for control of vertigo in unilateral Meniere's disease: A prospective, double-blind, randomized, placebo-controlled trial. Acta oto-laryngologica. 2008;**128**(8):876-880

[27] Bremer HG, Van Rooy I, Pullens B, Colijn C, Stegeman I, Van der Zaag-Loonen HJ, Bruintjes TD. Intratympanic gentamicin treatment for Ménière's disease: A randomized, double-blind, placebo-controlled trial on dose efficacy-results of a prematurely ended study. Trials. 2014;**15**(1):1

[28] Pullens B, van Benthem PP. Intratympanic gentamicin for Ménière's disease or syndrome. Cochrane Database of Systematic Reviews 2011, Issue 3. Art. No.: CD008234. DOI: 10.1002/14651858.CD008234.pub2. 1-13.

[29] Sharon JD, Trevino C, Schubert MC, Carey JP. Treatment of Meniere's disease. Current Treatment Options in Neurology. 2015;**17**(4):1-16

[30] Sun GH, et al. Analysis of hearing preservation after endolymphatic mastoid sac surgery for Meniere's disease. The Laryngoscope. 2010;**120**(3):591-597

[31] Sajjadi H, Paparella MM. Meniere's disease. Lancet. 2008;**372**:406-414

[32] Ghossaini, Soha N, Wazen JJ. An update on the surgical treatment of Ménière's diseases. Journal of the American Academy of Audiology. 2006;**17**(1):38-44

[33] Silverstein H, Norrell H, Rosenberg S. The resurrection of vestibular neurectomy: A 10-year experience with 115 cases. Journal of Neurosurgery. 1990;**72**:533-539

[34] Glasscock III ME, Thedinger BA, Cueva RA, Jackson CG. An analysis of the retrolabyrinthine vs. the retrosigmoid vestibular nerve section. Journal of Otolaryngology – Head & Neck Surgery. 1991;**104**:88-95

[35] McKenna MJ, Nadol Jr JB, Ojemann RG, Halpin C. Vestibular neurectomy: Retrosigmoid-intracanalicular versus retrolabyrinthine approach. The American Journal of Otology. 1996;**17**(2):253-258

[36] Molony TB. Decision making in vestibular neurectomy. The American Journal of Otology. 1996;**17**:421-424

[37] Rosenberg SI. Vestibular surgery for Ménière's disease in the elderly: A review of techniques and indications. Ear, Nose & Throat Journal. 1999;**78**:443-446

[38] Shah S, Ignatius A, Ahsan S. It is 2015: What are the best diagnostic and treatment options for Ménière's disease? World Journal of Otorhinolaryngology. 2016;**6**(1):1-12

[39] Zwolan TA, Shepard NT, Niparko JK. Labyrinthectomy with cochlear implantation. The American Journal of Otology. 1993;**14**:220-203

[40] Heywood RL. Simultaneous cochlear implantation and labyrinthectomy for advanced Ménière's disease. The Journal of Laryngology & Otology. 2016;**130**(2):204-206

[41] Inglestadt S, Ivarsson A, Tjernstron O. Immediate relief of symptoms during acute attacks of Meneire's disease using a pressure chamber. Acta Otolaryngol 1976;**82**:368-378

[42] Densert B, Arlinger S, Odkvist L, et al. Effects of middle ear pressure changes on the electrocochleographic recordings in patients with Meniere's disease. Presented at the 4th International Symposium on Meniere's Disease, Paris, France: Elsevier; 1999

[43] Ahsan SF, Standring R, Wang Y. Systematic review and meta-analysis of Meniett therapy for Meniere's disease. The Laryngoscope. 2015;**125**(1):203-208

[44] Gottshall KR, et al. Vestibular rehab: The role of vestibular rehabilitation in the treatment of Meniere's disease. Otolaryngology – Head and Neck Surgery. 2005;**133**(3):326-328

Chapter 13

Intratympanic Drug Delivery for Tinnitus Treatment

Monique Antunes De Souza Chelminski Barreto,
Alleluia Lima Losno Ledesma,
Marlene Escher Boger and
Carlos Augusto Costa Pires De Oliveira

Additional information is available at the end of the chapter

http://dx.doi.org/10.5772/intechopen.69664

Abstract

Objective: The aim of the study to evaluate the effectiveness of oral and injection intratympanic methylprednisolone to treat acute tinnitus associated with idiopathic sudden sensorineural hearing loss.

Study design: Analytical, prospective and longitudinal study.

Setting: Brasilia Institute of Otorhinolaryngology.

Subjects and methods: Twenty-three subjects with acute tinnitus and idiopathic sudden sensorineural hearing loss, 13 treated with oral steroids only (Group 1) and 10 treated with methylprednisolone intratympanic injection as rescue therapy (Group 2), and evaluated by audiometry, otoacoustic emission, tinnitus handicap inventory (THI) and visual analog scale (VAS) to assess the degree of tinnitus annoyance, before treatment and after 3 months.

Results: The annoyance due to tinnitus resulted in a mean VAS of 7.69 in the beginning of treatment and 5.15 3 months after treatment (Group 1), and 8.30 at the beginning and 6.00 3 months later (Group 2). In THI, average was 64.77 points at the beginning of treatment and 49.92 points 3 months later (Group 1) and 72.20 points at the beginning and 51.60 points after 3 months (Group 2). The results of audiometry and otoacoustic emissions showed significant improvement in both groups with significant differences intragroups before and after, but not between the groups.

Conclusion: The results suggest that both oral and injection intratympanic methylprednisolone are effective treatment for acute tinnitus associated with idiopathic sudden sensorineural hearing loss in these patients.

Keywords: tinnitus, idiopathic sudden sensorineural hearing loss, treatment, intratympanic, corticosteroids

INTECH
open science | open minds

© 2017 The Author(s). Licensee InTech. This chapter is distributed under the terms of the Creative Commons Attribution License (http://creativecommons.org/licenses/by/3.0), which permits unrestricted use, distribution, and reproduction in any medium, provided the original work is properly cited.

1. Introduction

Tinnitus is a complex disorder and is presented as a hearing sensation, which is not associated with an external sound stimulus [1]. It probably arises initially in the cochlea and later reaches higher structures of the auditory system where it becomes sometimes very annoying (severe disabling tinnitus—SDT).

One study showed 10 patients with "predominantly cochlear tinnitus" treated using intratympanic dexamethasone injections and described 5 patients with tinnitus control for at least 1 year [2]. They did not use a control group.

The effectiveness of intratympanic dexamethasone injections as a treatment for SDT was studied [3]. A control group was treated with saline solution and a study group with dexamethasone solution, both using intratympanic injections. There was no statistic significant difference between saline and dexamethasone solution regarding tinnitus improvement measured with visual analog scale (VAS). They concluded that intratympanic injections of steroids are not effective for the treatment of chronic SDT.

For acute tinnitus, interventions such as intratympanic AM-101 (a cochlear N-methyl-D-aspartate receptor antagonist) were tested. However, there is insufficient evidence to support the safety and efficacy of this intervention [4]. A second phase study was carried out, randomized, and placebo controlled using AM-101 intratympanic injections and concluded that the duration of symptoms affected the cure rate of intratympanic therapy for acute subjective tinnitus [5].

The management of subjective tinnitus associated with idiopathic sudden sensorineural hearing loss (ISSHL) includes oral, intravenous, and/or intratympanic administration of corticosteroids as initial therapy [6]. Intratympanic corticosteroids were effective for the treatment of idiopathic sudden sensorineural hearing loss (ISSHL) in controlled trials when used as primary therapy [7] or as rescue therapy after failure of initial oral steroids therapy [6].

The sudden sensorineural hearing loss (SSHL) is a hearing loss of at least 30 dB at three consecutive frequencies occurring in the period of 3 days or less [8] may occur in frequencies and intensities varying from a mild hearing loss to a total loss of hearing [9, 10].

SSHL is often accompanied by tinnitus and there are few theories trying to explain its mechanism. One of them associates this symptom to a maladaptive attempt at cortical reorganization process due to peripheral deafferentation [7].

Many of these patients with tinnitus and SHL remain with residual buzz even if the treatment for SHL has been effective. The treatment of sudden sensorineural hearing loss is based on its etiology. In idiopathic sudden sensorineural hearing loss (ISSHL), the oral corticosteroids are widely used, although the supporting evidence is weak. Injection intratympanic dexamethasone has been tried in patients with idiopathic sudden sensorineural hearing loss because it provides a high concentration of steroids in the labyrinth in animal models [8]. In addition, there are several advantages to intratympanic treatment. The procedure is well tolerated, relatively easy to perform as outpatient. Most patients understand the concept of intratympanic treatment and easily accept this therapy [3].

The questions we try to ask in this paper are as follows:

1. Are steroids intratympanic injections effective in the treatment of acute tinnitus? (As in ISSHL).

2. If so, what explains the fact it is not effective to treat chronic SDT?

2. Methods

The study protocol and procedures were approved by the Research Ethics Committee (REC) University of Brasilia (Opinion number 132/2012). All patients received information about the risks and expectations of therapy and signed a free informed consent form (FICF) accepting their participation in the study.

This is an analytical, prospective and longitudinal study, and the data were analyzed between January (2014) and June (2015).

Patients with middle ear diseases; presence of air type tympanogram, Ad, Ar, B, or C; prior ear surgery; signs of acute or chronic otitis media; history of Meniere's syndrome or fluctuating hearing; and history of prior sensorineural hearing loss were excluded (**Figure 1**).

From the initial sample of 38 patients with acute tinnitus and idiopathic sudden hearing loss, 23 were enrolled, 13 in the oral steroid therapy group (Group 1/oral therapy) and 10 in the intratympanic corticosteroids group after failure of oral therapy (Group 2/rescue therapy).

Tinnitus handicap inventory (THI) [11] and visual analog scale (VAS) were used for evaluation of tinnitus annoyance. For audiological assessment, tonal and vocal audiometry were used. (Diagnostic audiometer Madson Itera II) and for distortion products otoacoustic emission (DPOAE) measurements OtoRead Portable Interacoustic device was used.

A detailed clinical history was taken, followed by an otoneurological examination and audiological assessment by tonal and vocal audiometry. DPOAE measurements and application of THI [11] and VAS were carried out before onset of therapy and 3 months later [6].

All patients underwent pure-tone audiometry (PTA) and speech audiometry carried out by the same audiologist before and after treatment. The mean was calculated based on pure-tone average at 500, 1000, 2000, and 4000 Hz [12].

For DPOAEs, primary tones f1 and f2 were presented at 55 and 65 dBSPL (sound pressure levels). The f2/f1 ratio was kept at approximately 1.2. The levels of the DPOAE at 2fi–f2 were recorded in four different frequencies (ranging between 2000 and 5000 Hz), DP-gram showed DP1 level (dB) and DP1 signal-to-noise ratio (dB).

All patients were treated with systemic oral therapy according to the local protocol (1 mg/kg/day prednisolone for 10 days, followed by decreasing doses thereafter). Next, rescue therapy with intratympanic methylprednisolone was offered after systemic therapy failed and no improvements were demonstrated audiometrically in 10 patients (Group 2).

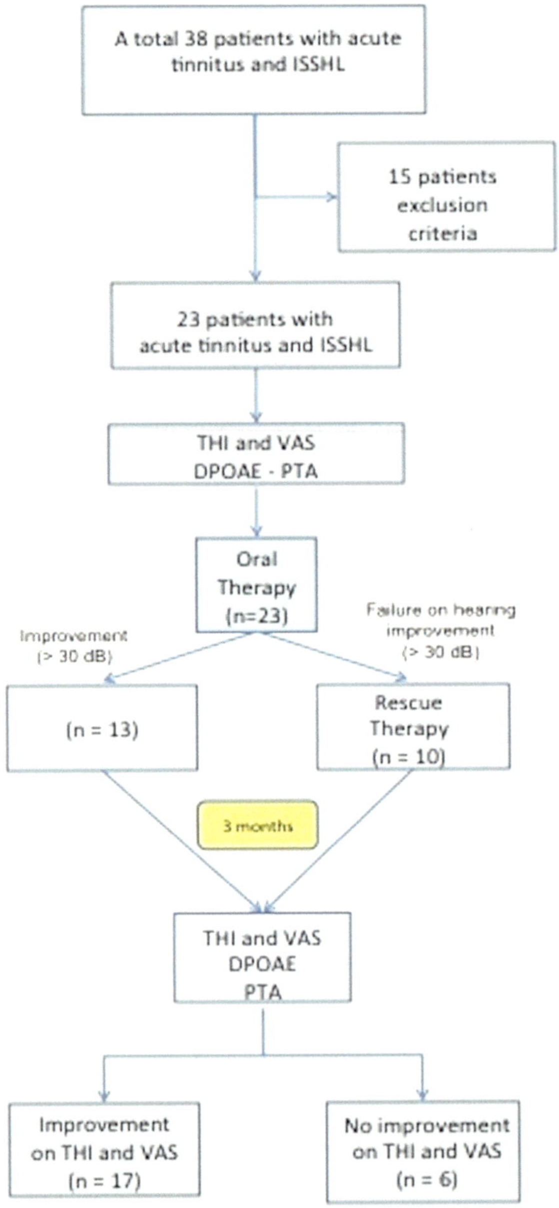

Figure 1. Schematic diagram.

Initially, EMLA cream was applied (AstraZeneca, Wilmington DE) for topical anesthesia in the external auditory canal and the tympanic membrane and left for 30–45 minutes. Then, the patient's head was placed at 45° in the direction of the affected ear. A solution of 40 mg of methylprednisolone/ml was warmed to body temperature. About 0.3–0.5 ml of the solution was injected into the middle ear; two holes were made with the application of needle (Gelco N.22), one just below the umbo (where the drug was administered) and another in the upper posterior region (vent). After intratympanic application of the steroid, the patient remained in the injection position with head turned 45° for 30 minutes to maximize exposure of the round window membrane to the solution and were applied three injections every 48 hours.

The criteria for defining successful recovery after therapy vary in the literature on intratympanic therapy. The hearing recovery was analyzed in three categories: (A) complete recovery when there was improvement ≥ 30 dBHL (hearing loss) in the affected frequencies; (B) partial recovery, when there was improvement ≥ 10 dBHL and ≤ 30 dBHL in the affected frequencies; (C) no recovery when there is an improvement of ≤ 9 dBHL [13]. Failure of oral prednisolone therapy was absence of improvement, as just described, after 14 days of treatment [14].

All patients answered the THI [11] and the VAS to assess quantitatively and qualitatively the therapeutic response in relation to tinnitus. In the VAS, score ranges from 1 to 10, where 10 represents the highest degree of tinnitus severity. Scores measured the intensity and discomfort of tinnitus. Two points in the VAS were considered significant change [3]. The THI questionnaire was considered improved when there was change of category of tinnitus severity in the following scale: Grade 1 negligible (0–16), Grade 2 light (18–36), Grade 3 moderate (38–56), Grade 4 severe (58–76), and Grade 5 catastrophic (78–100) [11].

The average posttreatment for some measures were compared between types of treatment (oral therapy and intratympanic corticosteroids after failure of oral therapy) using an analysis of covariance model (ANCOVA). In the ANCOVA model, the measurement obtained after treatment was considered the dependent variable, the type of treatment as the independent variable and the measures at baseline as the covariate. Mean comparisons were made with the intragroup test employing Student *t*-test for paired samples. Note that $p < 0.05$ was considered significant. The analysis was performed using SAS v 9.4 (SAS Institute, Inc., 2012).

3. Results

There were 23 subjects in the total, 13 subjects (6 female and 7 male, mean age = 38.30 years) in the oral steroid therapy (Group 1) and 10 subjects (7 female and 3 male, mean age = 47.40 years) in the intratympanic corticosteroids after failure of oral therapy (Group 2).

The average total score in THI before in Group 1 ($n = 13$) was 64.77 points, and after oral therapy, it was 45.90 points. The mean of the THI score before intratympanic corticosteroids after failure of oral therapy (Group 2) ($n = 10$) was 72.20 points and 47.73 points after (**Figure 2**). The mean VAS value in Group 1 was 7.69 points before and 5.30 points after therapy. The average value in VAS for the Group 2 was 8.30 points before and 5.81 points after therapy (**Figure 3**). THI and VAS averages showed a significant decrease when comparing the values before and after treatment intragroups ($p < 0.05$), whereas the analysis between groups was not statistically different.

In pure tone audiometry, we found the average of 74.23 dB (Group 1) before and 59.69 dB after therapy and 86.50 dB before and 51.91 dB after therapy (Group 2; **Figure 4**). A significant decrease in pure tone thresholds was found when comparing the values before and after treatment intragroups ($p < 0.05$), whereas the analysis between groups was not statistically different.

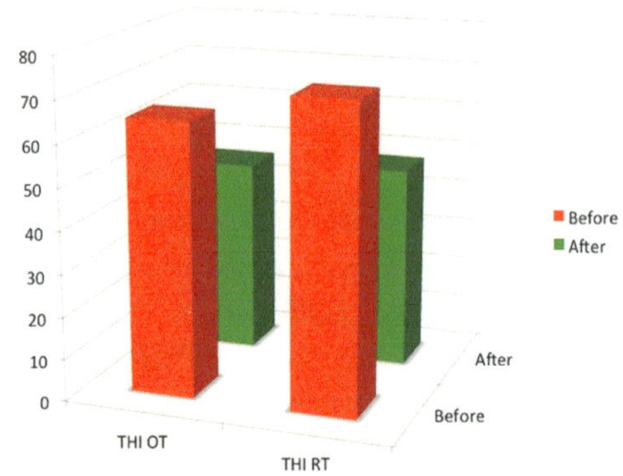

Figure 2. THI results before and after treatment.

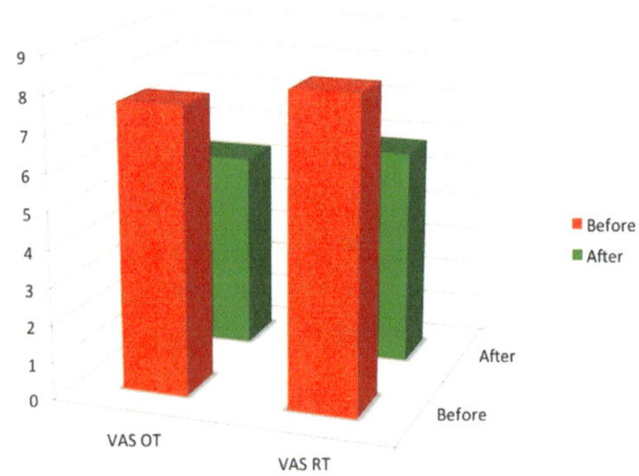

Figure 3. VAS results before and after treatment.

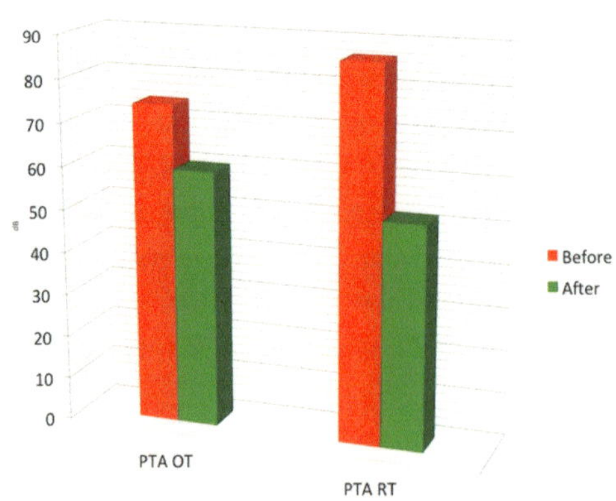

Figure 4. PTA results before and after treatment.

In the DPOAE test, we found in Group 1 the following amplitude values before and after therapy: for frequencies of 2 KHz: −10.08 and −1.69 dB; 3 KHz: −9.77 and −1.85 dB; 4 KHz: −10.92 and −5.08 dB; and 5 KHz: −10.69 and −2.85 dB. As for Group 2, the following amplitude values were obtained before and after treatment, respectively: 2 KHz: −12.30 and −3.90 dB; 3 KHz: −12.00 and −7.10 dB; 4 KHz: −11.30 and −6.10 dB, and 5 KHz: −12.60 and −4.40 dB (**Figure 5**).

As for the S/N ratio, the following values were obtained in Group 1 before and after therapy, for each frequency tested: 2 KHz: 2.77 and 8.38 dB; 3 KHz: 2.23 and 8.69; 4 KHz: 0.00 and 7.85 dB, and 5 KHz: 1.23 and 8.08 dB (**Figure 6**). We found a significant decrease when comparing the amplitude values before and after treatment intragroups ($p < 0.05$) in the four analyzed frequencies (2, 3, 4, and 5 KHz), while the analysis between groups did not show statistical difference.

The S/N ratios were as follows before and after treatment, respectively: 2 KHz: 0.00 and 7.10 dB; 3 KHz: 0.50 and 7.10 dB; 4 KHz: 1.00 and 4.30 dB, and 5 KHz: −0.70 and 4.50 dB (**Figure 6**). There was decrease when comparing signal/noise values before and after treatment intragroups ($p < 0.05$) in four analyzed frequencies (2 and 5 KHz), while the analysis between groups was not statistically different.

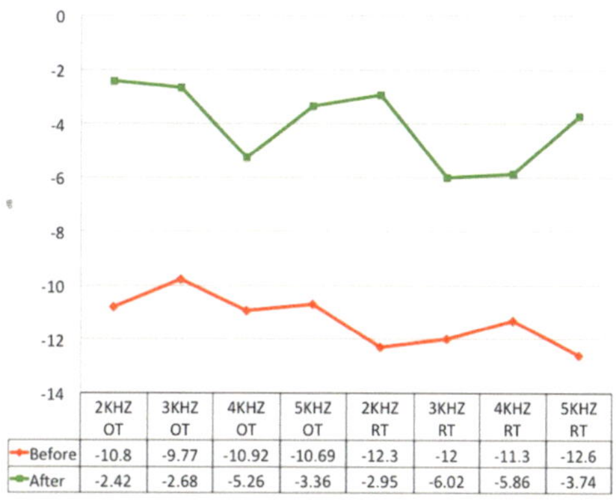
0
-2
-4
-6
-8
-10
-12
-14
2KHZ OT
3KHZ OT
4KHZ OT
5KHZ OT
2KHZ RT
3KHZ RT
4KHZ RT
5KHZ RT
Before -10.8 -9.77 -10.92 -10.69 -12.3 -12 -11.3 -12.6
After -2.42 -2.68 -5.26 -3.36 -2.95 -6.02 -5.86 -3.74

Figure 5. Amplitude results before and after treatment.

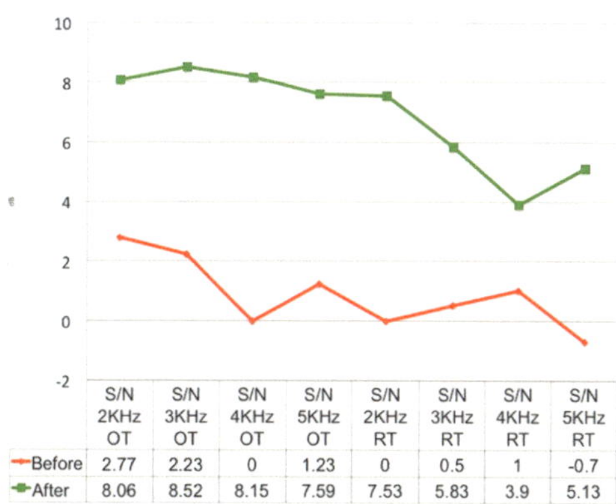

Figure 6. Signal/noise results before and after treatment.

4. Discussion

In this study, the treatment of sudden deafness and acute tinnitus with intratympanic corticosteroids after failure of oral therapy (rescue) was effective. The findings were consistent with the study in which the THI and VAS scores were significantly reduced after intratympanic steroids injections, and it was concluded that these scores were useful for assessing tinnitus patients, as well as it [15].

The intratympanic therapy is currently in use for ISSHL, Meniere's disease, tinnitus associated with these disorders and idiopathic tinnitus [15]. In previous studies, positive results of intratympanic steroids injections were reported for chronic subjective tinnitus [2, 16, 17], but they did not use the control group. Statistic significant difference between saline and dexamethasone solution when a control group was used regarding tinnitus improvement measured with visual analog scale (VAS).

A systematic review was conducted to determine the efficacy of intratympanic steroids treatment. It emphasized that this treatment should be considered as an adjuvant one in sudden deafness [18] consistent with the findings of this study.

The analysis of the characteristics of sudden deafness in 105 patients pointed out that there are individual differences in clinical characteristics between patients with tinnitus and ISSHL hindering a single treatment line [19]. We emphasize that both groups of this study were homogeneous, showing no statistical difference in age, sex, and affected ear.

By examining variables such as gender, age, and laterality in relation to changes in the level of tinnitus after the start of ISSHL, our results corroborate previous studies in which patients requiring rescue therapy were those in which oral therapy had not been sufficient to improve the hearing thresholds. Some patients improved hearing thresholds but remained with residual tinnitus [20].

Overall good results were reported in 77% of patients with tinnitus and various diseases immediately after the intratympanic dexamethasone treatment [21] and found that the best results of intratympanic therapy for tinnitus are obtained in patients with a shorter duration of tinnitus, especially when treatment was initiated within 3 months of symptom onset [17]. The effectiveness of intratympanic injection of prednisolone or dexamethasone to treat subjective tinnitus was reported to be 48.6 and 37.5%, respectively [22].

Similar results were found by other researchers that recommended intratympanic therapy as a possible option in the treatment of tinnitus to a certain group of patients [3, 23]. No difference in results was observed in patients between 3 and 6 months after treatment [23].

The shorter the period from onset of sudden deafness to the start of intratympanic treatment with dexamethasone, the greater the improvement in tinnitus that could be expected after treatment [24]. There is no significant difference after 3 months [6].

In this study, we chose to use intratympanic corticosteroid as rescue after failure of oral corticosteroids. We found that this association was particularly effective in relation to tinnitus. In Group 2, VAS and THI showed a significant reduction of tinnitus annoyance after intratympanic steroids therapy. Probably, these results are due to the fact that the rescue treatment was initiated immediately after the oral treatment did not show the desired results.

It is significant the correlation between the degree of hearing recovery and subjective improvement of tinnitus after treatment. It was suggested that the hearing improvement may be a prognostic factor for tinnitus improvement, but the presence of tinnitus was not a prognostic factor for the recovery of hearing [25]. These findings are similar to those of the present study.

In this study, Group 2 had increase in the amplitude of DPOAE in all frequencies. There are studies in the literature that demonstrate a prognostic role for OAEs in the ISSHL [21, 26]. Other studies do not agree with this [27, 28].

The DPOAE is detectable in three of five patients whose hearing had significantly improved. It is suggested that the presence of DPOAE can be a useful prognostic factor that positively correlates with the recovery of the SHL [29].

It is reported a significant increase in the amplitude of DPOAE among patients who regained their hearing and also found significant correlations between improvement in DPOAE and improved hearing. It was stated that the presence of DPOAE predicted improvement in hearing [28, 30]. Our study is in agreement with these previous studies.

The detection of OAE during the first 15 days after starting treatment, even with no improvement in hearing, would suggest the high sensitivity of this test to detect improvement changes in the activity of outer hair cells [31].

The sudden deafness factors that predict a favorable prognosis are still controversial. Clinical recovery was estimated by the difference between the audiometric results on admission and the audiometric results 10 days later. Only two factors were significantly associated with improved hearing: tinnitus ($p < 0.04$) and the configuration of ascending audiometric curve at admission ($p < 0.045$) [32]. In this study, most subjects had flat audiometric curve.

Tinnitus was cured in 43 of 114 patients (37.7%) within 3 months. In our study, THI was significantly reduced after intratympanic dexamethasone, and this cure rate was significantly higher in patients with symptoms lasting 2 weeks or less. The authors concluded that the duration of symptoms affected the intratympanic dexamethasone cure rate for acute subjective tinnitus [33].

The feeling of ear fullness and tinnitus in ISSHL was compared in one study that found they were primarily associated with poorer hearing thresholds at high frequencies. They concluded that tinnitus is probably originated in the region where the hair cells are damaged [34]. Steroid intratympanic therapy for acute tinnitus was found effective. SSHL patients were excluded from that study. Our study is about ISSNHL patients with tinnitus that is necessarily acute.

Steroids were likewise effective for these patients. Probably, the short time from onset of tinnitus is the determinant factor to predict the effectiveness of steroids therapy.

Our study has some limitations that should be pointed out: we did not have a control group, as this group would be composed of patients who failed on oral therapy and were not treated with rescue therapy, which would not be correct from the point of view ethics and the number of patients is small in preliminary studies. Therefore, to confirm our results, we should consider a larger number of patients in future studies.

5. Conclusions

Our results as well as other studies seem to point out to the effectiveness of steroids for the treatment of acute tinnitus. Both oral and intratympanic steroids were effective in our study. Intratympanic steroids improved tinnitus further in patients that did not respond well to oral steroids. The higher concentration of steroids in inner ear fluids after intratympanic injection probably explains this result.

Why steroids are effective to treat acute tinnitus and not to treat chronic tinnitus? We believe tinnitus start in the cochlea almost always. Later the cochlea lesion causes changes in central pathways that in some patients make the symptom permanent and extremely annoying-severe disabling tinnitus (SDT) [2]. If tinnitus is treated before it sets foot in the central pathways (acute tinnitus), steroid therapy is effective.

Author details

Monique Antunes De Souza Chelminski Barreto*, Alleluia Lima Losno Ledesma, Marlene Escher Boger and Carlos Augusto Costa Pires De Oliveira

*Address all correspondence to: nikebarr@hotmail.com

University of Brasilia, Brasília, Brazil

References

[1] Eggermont JJ. Pathophysiology of tinnitus. Progress in Brain Research. 2007;**166**:19-36

[2] Shulman A, Goldstein B. Intratympanic drug therapy with steroids for tinnitus control. The International Tinnitus Journal. 2000;**6**:10-20

[3] Araujo MFS, Oliveira CA, Bahmad Jr F. Intratympanic dexamethasone injections as a treatment for severe, disabling tinnitus. Does it work? Head and Neck Surgery. 2005;**131**:113-117

[4] Muehlmeir G, Biesinger E, Maier H. Safety of intratympanic injection of AM-101 in patients with acute inner ear tinnitus. Audiology and Neurotology. 2011;**16**:388-397

[5] Heyning PV, Muehlmeir G, Cox T, Lisowska G, et al. Efficacy and safety of AM-101 in the treatment of acute inner ear tinnitus a double-blind, randomized, placebo-controlled phase II study. Otology & Neurotology. 2014;**35**:589-597

[6] Stachler RJ, Chandrasekhar SS, Archer SM, Rosenfeld RM, et al. Clinical practice guideline: Sudden hearing loss. Otolaryngology Head and Neck Surgery. 2012;**146**:S1-S35

[7] Rauch SD, Halpin CF, Antonielle PJ, Babu S, et al. Oral vs intratympanic corticosteroid therapy for idiopathic sudden sensorineural hearing loss. The Journal of the American Medical Association. 2011;**305**:2071-2079

[8] Schreiber BE, Charlotte A, Dorian OH, Linda ML. Sudden sensorineural hearing loss. The Lancet. 2010;**375**:1203-1211

[9] Maia RA, Cahali S. Surdez súbita. Brazilian Journal of Otorhinolaryngology. 2004;**70**: 238-248

[10] Penido NO, Ramos HVL, Barros FA, Cruz OLM, et al. Clinical and etiological factors and evolution of hearing in sudden deafness. Brazilian Journal of Otorhinolaryngology. 2005;**71**:633-638

[11] Ferreira PEA, Cunha F, Onishi ET, Branco-Barreiro FCA, et al. Tinnitus handicap inventory: Cultural adaptation to Brazilian. Pró-Fono R Atual Cient. 2005;**17**:303-310

[12] Halpin CF, Shi H, Reda D, Antonelli PJ, et al. Audiology in the sudden hearing loss: Clinical trial. Otology & Neurotology. 2012;**33**(6):907-911

[13] Nemati S, Naghavi SE, Kazemnejad E, Banan R. Otoacoustic emissions in sudden sensorineural hearing loss: Changes of measures with treatment. Iranian Journal of Otorhinolaringology. 2011;**23**(1):37-44

[14] Raymundo IT, Bahmad FJr, Barros Filho JB, Pinheiro TG, et al. Intratympanic methylprednisolone as rescue therapy in sudden sensorineural hearing loss. Brazilian Journal of Otorhinolaryngology. 2010;**76**:499-509

[15] Tinnitus assessment by THI and VAS in patients with sudden sensorineural hearing loss Wang, P., et al., Lin chuang er bi yan hou tou jing wai ke za zhi = Journal of clinical otorhinolaryngology, head, and neck surgery, 2014;28(22): p. 1777-9

[16] Dodson KM, Sismanis A. Intratympanic perfusion for the treatment of tinnitus. Otolaryngologic Clinics of North America. 2004;**37**:991-1000

[17] Cesarani A, Capobianco S, Soi D, Giuliano DA, et al. Intratympanic dexamethasone treatment for control of subjective idiophatic tinnitus: Our clinical experience. The International Tinnitus Journal. 2002;**8**:111-113

[18] Lavigne P, Lavigne F, Saliba I. Intratympanic corticosteroids injections: A systematic review of literature. European Archives of Otorhinolaryngology. 2015;**23**:1-8

[19] The study of clinical characteristics of sudden sensorineural hearing loss patients with tinnitus Li, Q., et al., Lin chuang er bi yan hou tou jing wai ke za zhi = Journal of clinical otorhinolaryngology, head, and neck surgery, 2015;29(1): p. 57-60

[20] Michiba T, Kitahara T, Hikita-Watanabe N, Fukushima M, et al. Residual tinnitus after the medical treatment of sudden deafness. Auris Nasus Larynx. 2013;**40**:162-166

[21] Sakashita T, Minowa Y, Hachikawa K. Evoked otoacoustic emissions from ears with idiopathic sudden deafness. Acta Otolaryngologica Supplementum. 1991;**486**:66-72

[22] She W, Dai Y, Du X, Chen F, et al. Treatment of subjective tinnitus: A comparative clinical study of intratympanic steroid injection vs. oral carbamazepine. Medical Science Monitor. 2009;**15**:35-39

[23] Choi SJ, Lee JB, Lim HJ, In SM, et al. Intratympanic dexamethasone injection for refractory tinnitus: Prospective placebo-controlled study. Laryngoscope. 2013;**123**(11):2817-2822

[24] Yoshida T, Teranishi M, Iwata T, Otake H, et al. Intratympanic injection of dexamethasone for treatment of tinnitus in patients with sudden sensorineural hearing loss. Audiol Research. 2012;**2**(1):4-7

[25] Rah YC, Park KT, Yi YJ, Seok J, et al. Successful treatment of sudden sensorineural hearing loss assures improvement of accompanying tinnitus. The Laryngoscope. 2015;**125**:1433-1437

[26] Ishida IM, Sugiura M, Teranishi M, Katayama M, et al. Otoacoustic emissions, ear fullness and tinnitus in the recovery course of sudden deafness. Auris Nasus Larynx. 2008;**35**:41-46

[27] Canale A, Lacilla M, Giordano C, De Sanctis A, et al. The prognostic value of the otoacoustic emission test in low frequency sudden hearing loss. European Archives of Otorhinolaryngology. 2005;**262**:208-212

[28] Hoth S. On a possible prognostic value of otoacoustic emissions: A study on patients with sudden hearing loss. European Archives of Otorhinolaryngology. 2006;**262**(3):217-224

[29] Schweinfurth JM, Cacace AT, Parnes SM. Clinical applications of otoacoustic emissions in sudden hearing loss. Laryngoscope. 1997;**107**:1457-1463

[30] Chao TK, Chen THH. Distortion product otoacoustic emissions as a prognostic factor for idiopathic sudden sensorineural hearing loss. Audiology and Neurotology. 2006;**11**:331-338

[31] Shupak A, Zeidan R, Shemesh R. Otoacoustic emissions in the prediction of sudden sensorineural hearing loss outcome. Otology & Neurotology. 2014;**10**:1-7

[32] Ben-David J, Luntz M, Magamsa I, Fradis M, et al. Tinnitus as a prognostic sign in idiopathic sudden sensorineural hearing loss. The International Tinnitus Journal. 2001;**7**(1):62-64

[33] An YH, Kyu KK, Kwak MY, Yoon SW, et al. Prognostic factors for the outcomes of intratympanic dexamethasone in the treatment of acute subjective tinnitus. Otology & Neurotology. 2014;**35**:1330-1337

[34] Sakata T, Esaki Y, Yamano T, Sueta N, et al. A comparison between the feeling of ear fullness and tinnitus in acute sensorineural hearing loss. International Journal of Audiology. 2008;**47**(3):134-140

Chapter 14

Intratympanic Steroid Treatment in Méniére Disease

Fatih Oghan, Ibrahim Erdim, Metin Çeliker,
Muhammet Fatih Topuz, Ahmet Uluat,
Onur Erdogan and Sinan Aksoy

Additional information is available at the end of the chapter

http://dx.doi.org/10.5772/intechopen.69665

Abstract

Méniére disease (MD) is characterized by vertigo attacks, hearing loss, tinnitus, and aural fullness. Although the exact treatment of MD is lacking, several treatment options including conservative, medical, and surgical aim to control symptoms. Recently, an increasingly used treatment method called intratympanic steroid (ITS) treatment is applied to patients suffering from MD. In which step the ITS takes part for MD treatment protocol is not certain. But common wisdom is that ITS can be used in patients with intractable MD to conservative and medical treatment before applying intratympanic gentamicin and surgical treatments.

Keywords: Méniére Disease, Steroid Treatment, Vertigo

1. Introduction

Méniére disease (MD) is characterized by vertigo attacks, hearing loss, tinnitus, and aural fullness. Several treatment options include conservative, medical, and surgical aims to control symptoms. Recently, an increasingly used treatment method called intratympanic steroid (ITS) treatment is applied to patients suffering from MD. In this chapter, we mention this alternative treatment option.

2. Pathophysiology

After Mc Cabe's report on auto-immune depended on sensorineural hearing loss in 1979, immunological mechanisms about inner ear pathologies started to be investigated [1]. Many

INTECH
open science | open minds

© 2017 The Author(s). Licensee InTech. This chapter is distributed under the terms of the Creative Commons Attribution License (http://creativecommons.org/licenses/by/3.0), which permits unrestricted use, distribution, and reproduction in any medium, provided the original work is properly cited. (cc) BY

studies showed that MD is an immune system-related disease. Autoantibody for the Raf-1 protein in the membranous labyrinth is found in patients with MD [2]. Elevated IgG immune complexes, auto-immune response to type II collagen, and focal inflammation with intraepithelial invasion caused by mononuclear cells are shown in endolymphatic sac. This phenomenon is also called "endolymphatic sacitis" [3, 4].

Rarey and Curtis found glycocorticoid receptors on the cochlea and vestibule (especially on the spiral ligament) [5]. Lohuis also showed cell atrophy on stria vascularis after adrenal steroid defects [6]. Glycocorticoid receptors are also found in the lateral wall of cochlea, organ of Corti, modiolus, vestibule, and stria vascularis [7].

It is already shown that steroids regulate inner ear fluid balance with potassium transport channels by mineralocorticoid receptor genes and aquaporin regulation [8, 9]. Cochlear blood flow is also positively affected by topical steroid application [10, 11].

According to these information and steroids' anti-inflammatory/immunosuppressive effects, we can say that ITS treatment is helpful for MD control.

3. Intratympanic steroid injection protocol

Procedure is done under operation microscope. Head is turned 45° to the opposite side. EMLA® 5% cream (lidocaine Hcl + prilocaine) or 88% phenol can be used for local anesthesia. Twenty-two or 25 gauge spinal needle can be used for injection. Myringotomy is made anterosuperior part of tympanic membrane to fill middle ear as long as possible. After intervention, the patient has to wait for 30–40 min as the head is turned 45° to the opposite side. During this time, the patient is requested not to speak and not to swallow as much as possible [12, 13].

4. Application features (steroid types, daily usage time, dosage, and time duration)

Despite many studies, there is no consensus for ITS application [14]. Three different types of steroids are used for ITS: hydrocortisone (short-acting), methylprednisolone (intermediate-acting), and dexamethasone (long-acting). Methylprednisolone and dexamethasone are generally preferred types in studies (**Table 1**). In some studies, it is claimed that methylprednisolone reaches inner ear tissues and fluids in shorter time (2 h), and maximum concentration continues by 6 h [4, 15]. However, other studies have claimed that dexamethasone reaches inner ear tissues and fluids in shorter time than methylprednisolone [15, 16].

Three different application ways are used for ITS: injection, ventilation tube, and perfusion with catheter. Daily intervention is recommended regardless of application ways. Methylprednisolone stays for 6 h at maximal concentration in blood and descends as basal level at 24 h. Dexamethasone also descends as basal level at 6 h. We recommend using a ventilation

Types of ITS in MD	Hydrocortisone	Methylprednisolone*	Dexamethasone*
Efficiency period	**Short-acting**	**Intermediate-acting**	**Long-acting**
Dosage		62.5 mg/ml, 3 weeks [3]	4 mg/ml, three times with 3 days interval [14, 18]
			17.5 mg, 0.3–0.8 ml applied each day for 5 days [12]
			4 mg/cc, 4 weeks [13]
			24 mg/cc [20]
			0.20 mg/cc, five drops in each day for 3 months [19]

*Preferred steroid types in studies, ITS: intratympanic steroid, MD: Ménière disease.

Table 1. Types, efficiency period, and dosage of ITS using in MD.

tube or catheter application for daily intervention that provides less patient pain and prevents time lost for both doctor and patient [15, 17].

Both the dosing of the steroid types and the daily usage protocols are also different in the studies. Dexamethasone (4 mg/ml) is used for three times at 3 days interval in two studies [14, 18]. In another study, 17.5 mg dexamethasone in 0.3–0.8 ml was applied each day for 5 days [12]. Ventilation tube application was made toward posteroinferior cadrane to 20 patients with MD in another study. In that study, 1 mg/cc dexamethasone was distilled to 0.20 mg/cc with water. Five drops were applied to 20 patients in each day for 3 months (**Table 1**) [19]. Barr et al. administered 4 mg/cc dexamethasone for 4 weeks [13]. Hamid et al. applied 24 mg/cc dexamethasone (**Table 1**) [20]. Nathalie Gabra et al. used methylprednisolone (62.5 mg/ml) each week for 3 weeks (**Table 1**) [3]. The reason for not performing daily intervention in these studies is the difficulty of injection application way [14]. All studies mentioned earlier show that vertigo control rates get higher when drug concentration increases.

5. Advantages

Steroids are permeable to round window and across blood-labyrinthine barrier [13] so drug concentration in inner ear fluids (both perilymph and endolymph) is higher with ITS application than systemic administration [3, 13]. ITS application also prevents steroid side effects.

6. Disadvantages and side effects

Tympanic membrane perforation may occur after ITS. Its incidence seems low and changes between 0 and 5.1%. If the tympanic membrane perforation develops after ITS, it may recover or be permanent [12, 14, 18, 21]. To reduce the likelihood of development perforation, it needs attention to not penetrate tympanic membrane from thinned areas.

Pain and burn sensation in the ear and pharynx are other problems. These resolve approximately 0.5–1 h later. Mild dizziness and transient vertigo may be seen due to inner ear content concentration change [4, 13, 18].

7. Treatment effects

Patients with MD suffer from vertigo attacks, hearing loss, tinnitus, and aural fullness. Life is also unbearable during MD attacks. We mention each symptom recovering rate by ITS treatment in subsequent text (**Table 2**).

	Vertigo	Hearing loss	Tinnitus	Aural fullness	Quality of life
Albu et al. [14]	46% class A 21.2% class B 24.2% class C/D 3% class E	PTA: Pretreatment 57.4 ± 14.7 After 1 year 55.8 ± 15.5	THI: Pretreatment 28.6 ± 14.3 Posttreatment 23.5 ± 12.4	–	DHI: Pretreatment 53.2 ± 13.4 Posttreatment 40.7 ± 16.5
Casani et al. [18]	42.9% class A 17.9% class B 32.2% class C/D 7% class E/F	PTA: Pretreatment 66.6 ± 16.4 After 1 month 67.5 ± 17.7 After 1 year 67.1 ± 17.6 After 2 years 65.0 ± 18.7	–	–	–
Gabra and Saliba [3]	**Number of attack** Before therapy: 5.3 ± 6.41 After 0–6 months: therapy 1.4 ± 1.87 After 6–12 months: therapy 1.4 ± 1.87	PTA: Pretreatment 41.89 ± 14.92 After 1 yeary 49.51 ± 17.9	Decreased to: 78% at 0–6 months therapy 68% at 6–12 months therapy	Pretreatment: 95.2% Posttreatment: 65%	–
Paragache et al. [19]	85% class A 10% class C/D 5% class E/F	PTA:15% improved 10% dropped SDS:15% improved 85% same	10% recovery 60% improved	15% Disappeared 65% Improved	–
Ren et al. [12]	48.8% class A 20.9% class B 9.3% class C/D 20.9% class E	–	Disappeared 11.6% Decreased 48.8% Same 23.3% Improved 16.3%	16.7%: Disappeared 45.8%: Alleviated 35.7%: Intensive	–
Barr et al. [13]	At 3rd month of therapy: 52% class A At 6th month of therapy: 43% class A	At 6th month of therapy: An average loss of 2.7 dB	–	–	–

	Vertigo	Hearing loss	Tinnitus	Aural fullness	Quality of life
Garduño-Anaya et al. [22]	82% class A 18% class B	PTA: Pretreatment 55.7 After 2 years 53.4 SDS: Pretreatment 68.5% After 2 years 66.7%	THI: 61 pretreatment 22.3 at 2 years therapy GTS: 3.2 pretreatment 1.6 at 2 years therapy	48% subjective improvement	DHI: Pretreatment 68.7 Posttreatment 8.3

ITS: Intratympanic steroid, MD: Méniére disease, PTA: Pure tone average, SDS: Speech discrimination score, THI: Tinnitus Handicap Inventory, GTS: Grading of Tinnitus Severity, DHI: Dizziness Handicap Inventory.

Table 2. Symptom relief success of ITS on MD.

7.1. Vertigo

Vertigo control is generally reported according to the 1995 AAO-HNS guidelines or Sakata's criteria in the studies about ITS treatment.

Albu et al. investigated 66 patients with definite unilateral MD. Thirty-three of them received IT dexamethasone. Fourteen patients (46.6%) were free from vertigo attack (class A), seven patients (21.2%) had substantial control (class B), and eight patients (24.2%) had limited control (classes C and D) at 1-year follow-up. Vertigo control couldn't be obtained in one patient (class E). Failures were planned for intratympanic gentamicin (ITG), which did not benefit enough from the ITC [14].

In Casani et al.'s study, 12 patients (42.9%) had full vertigo control (class A), 5 patients (17.9%) had substantial control (class B), 9 patients (32.2%) had limited control (class C or D) despite 1 or 2 additional intratympanic dexamethasone (ITD). Two patients (7%) couldn't get vertigo control (class E or F) and were scheduled for ITG therapy [18].

In a study, Gabra and Saliba had evaluated the effect of intratympanic methylprednisolone and gentamicin injection on MD. In this study, the number of patient's vertigo attacks per month before ITS (for methylprednisolone) was 5.3 ± 6.41 (n = 42). In 0–6 months after the ITS, the number of attacks decreased to 2.3 ± 3.20 (n = 41). Finally, 6–12 months after ITS, attack frequency was 1.4 ± 1.87 (n = 27). In the first period after treatment, 41.5% of the patients achieved complete control of vertigo. In the second period after treatment, 48.1% of the patients achieved complete control of vertigo (P = 0.004). There was a statistically significant decrease in the number of vertigo attacks in the first period (P = 0.025) and no difference between the 0- to 6-month and 6- to 12-month periods after ITS (P = 0.95) [3].

Paragache et al. reported 85% (17 of 20 patients) control of vertigo with intratympanic dexamethasone therapy. Two patients (10%) had only limited control. One patient (5%) had worsening of vertigo during treatment [19].

Boleas-Aguirre et al. reported 91% "acceptable" vertigo control using 12 mg/ml dexamethasone. Most of the patients (63%) needed more than one series of treatment for achieving remission of MD [21].

Ren et al. reported complete control of vertigo in 21 of 43 patients (48.8%), substantial control in 9 patents (20.9%), limited control in 4 patients (9.3%), and no exact response in 9 patients (20.9%) with intratympanic dexamethasone injections for refractory MD after 18 months follow-up [12].

In a retrospective analysis of 17 intractable MD patients treated with ITD, short-term (after 6 months) and long-term (after 24 months) vertigo control rates were 94 and 81% [4].

Barrs's et al. reported that 21 patients with intractable MD underwent intratympanic injections of 4 mg/ml dexamethasone over a period of 4 weeks as an office procedure. Eleven (52%) of 21 patients were free for vertigo attack at the 3rd month of treatment. However, vertigo attacks relapsed in two patients and success rate decreased to 43% at the 6th month. At 1-year follow-up, six of remaining nine patients had no vertigo attack. Recurrent injections applied to five patients who responded at the beginning but repeated vertigo attacks later. Vertigo was controlled in three of those five patients. One patient got only one additional injection but two patients got multiple injections for each month up to 6 months [13].

In another prospective, randomized, double-blind study with a 2-year follow-up, the effect of five consecutive daily intratympanic injections of dexamethasone on 22 patients having definite MD was investigated. Complete control of vertigo (class A) was achieved in 9 of 11 patients (82%) and substantial control of vertigo (class B) in the remaining 2 patients (18%) [22].

In a retrospective study including 129 patients diagnosed with unilateral MD still having vertigo despite medical therapy, patient's satisfaction with vertigo attack control using ITD (12 mg/ml) was assessed. Vertigo control was obtained in 117 (91%) of 129 patients. One injection was enough for 48 patients (37%), two injections were needed for 26 patients (20%), three injections for 18 patients (14%), and four injections for 10 patients (8%). More than four injections were needed for 15 patients (21%). Ninety-six patients were followed for 2 years. Vertigo control was obtained in 87 (91%) patients with ITD. After 2 years, additional injection wasn't needed in 61 patients but repeated injections were required in 23 patients. Three patients requested ITG treatment because of repeated ITD injections [21].

Different vertigo control rates were given in studies mentioned earlier. This may be related to steroid type, concentration, time duration, and frequency of therapy. Also keep in mind that each drug has different personal effect.

7.2. Hearing loss

Sensorineural hearing loss is another symptom of MD. It may be transient or permanent. The success of any treatment about MD on hearing improvement is a change of 10 dB or more in pure tone average (PTA) or a change of 15% in speech discrimination score (SDS) according to 1995 AAO-HNS guidelines [3, 14, 18].

Paragache et al. observed hearing improvement in only three patients (15%) with two patients (10%) having a 20-dB improvement in threshold and one patient (5%) having a 10-dB improvement in threshold. In 10% of patients, the hearing level was observed to decrease. The speech discrimination score improved in three patients (15%). For the rest, the SDS remained the same with the intratympanic dexamethasone applications [19].

Albu et al. found the mean pretreatment PTA as 57.4 (standard deviation (SD), 14.7) with the intratympanic dexamethasone injection. After 12 months of therapy, the PTA values were 55.8 (SD, 15.5). Hearing was unchanged in 14 patients, improved in 4 patients and worsened in 12 patients. With reference to hearing outcomes, they had demonstrated that hearing conservation was only able to be maintained in patients reporting vertigo, which was well controlled. As previously stated [18], hearing loss is associated with the evolution of MD [14, 23].

Casani et al. found the mean pretreatment PTA as 66.6 (SD, 16.4). After 1 month with ITD injection, the PTA values changed on average to 67.5 (SD, 17.7). The mean PTA was 67.1 (SD, 17.6) at 1 year and 65.0 (SD, 18.7) at 2-year follow-up with the intratympanic ITD injection. No significant variations of SDS were observed during each follow-up period ($P > 0.05$) [18]. Hearing improved in 3 patients (10.7%) and did not worsen in 13 patients (46.4%). Vertigo was detected as class A and class B in those 16 patients. Hearing deterioration on PTA was more than 10 dB in remaining 10 patients who couldn't obtain vertigo control [18]. It pays attention that a correlation was found between hearing deterioration and vertigo attack persistence.

Gabra et al. found the mean PTA as 41.89 ± 14.92 dB before intratympanic methylprednisolone injection (ITM). There was a slight increase in PTA at 6 months. This was followed by an increase in PTA at 12 months after ITM, the mean PTA was 49.51 ± 17.9 dB. There was no statistically significant difference in the evolution from before to after treatment ($P = 0.456$ for the 0- to 6-month period and $P = 0.06$ for the 6- to 12-month period) [3]. In the first 0–6 months, the SDS decreased and remained stable in the second period. There was no statistically significant difference in the evolution of SDS after ITM [3].

Another retrospective analysis was conducted on 17 MD patients treated with ITM. Sixteen patients were followed up for more than 2 years. The PTA was 53 ± 14 dB before treatment, and 50 ± 16 dB at 6 months and 52 ± 20 dB at 24 months after ITM. Thus, a significant improvement in PTA after 6 months had returned to the pretreatment baseline after 2 years and there were no significant differences in clinical stage, based on hearing changes at the 6- and 24-month follow-up [4].

Garduño-Anaya et al. found the mean initial PTA as 55.7 dB and after receiving the ITD the mean PTA was 53.4 dB at 2-year follow-up. Only one patient's hearing (9%) improvement, 10 dB or more according to the 1995 AAO-HNS criteria, was considered to be clinically significant. One of 11 patients was demonstrated to have hearing deterioration of 10 dB at 2-year follow-up [22]. The mean SDS was 68.5% at the beginning of treatment and 66.7% after 2 years of ITD. According to 1995 AAO-HNS criteria, 15% or higher improvement on SDS was provided in two patients (18%). Only one (9%) of 11 patients got 15% or higher deterioration at 2 years follow-up. They reported a subjective improvement of 35% in hearing loss [22].

Kaplan et al. investigated 30 patients (20 women and 10 men, aged 28–85 years) with MD who underwent intratympanic dexamethasone perfusion. Six patients obtained 10 dB or higher improvement at PTA and six patients obtained 15% or higher improvement at SDS at short-term period (4 weeks after perfusion). Those patient numbers decreased to 5 and 2 at 12 months later, respectively [23].

Arriaga and Goldman demonstrated that only 33% of patients had hearing improvement, and 20% of patients had hearing deterioration after ITD with hyaluronan. However, Hillman et al. [24] reported 40% of patients who had hearing improvement after ITD [21].

7.3. Tinnitus

In Paragache et al.'s study, 2 patients (of 20, 10%) showed complete relief from tinnitus and tinnitus improved in 12 patients (60%) [19]. In Gabra et al.'s study, all patients suffered from tinnitus before ITM injections. Tinnitus rate decreased to 78% for 0–6 month period and 68% for 6–12 months period [3]. Tinnitus symptom disappeared in 5 (11.6%) of 43 patients, decreased in 21 (48.8%) patients, didn't change in 10 (23.3%) patients, and increased in 7 (16.3%) patients after ITD in Ren et al.'s study [12].

In a retrospective analysis of 17 intractable MD patients treated with ITM perfusion, 16 patients were followed up for more than 2 years. Tinnitus was controlled in three patients and improved in two patients at the 24-month follow-up, and patient without tinnitus worsened over this interval [4].

Another study measured tinnitus severity with "Tinnitus Handicap Inventory" score and the "Grading of Tinnitus Severity." Eleven patients with unilateral MD were treated with ITD. The initial mean handicap score was 61 and after receiving ITD was 22.3 at 2 years of follow-up. At 2 years of follow-up, a handicap score of 0 was found in 4 of 11 patients (36%) [22]. The initial "Grading of Tinnitus Severity" score was 3.2 and after receiving ITD injection was 1.6 at 2 years of follow-up. Grade 1 of the Grading of Tinnitus Severity (THI 0–16) at 2-year follow-up was achieved by 8 of 11 patients (72%). At 2-year follow-up, 1 of 11 patients (9%) in the dexamethasone group reported improvement of 100% and 1 other patient (9%) reported 90% improvement. Five of 11 patients (45%) reported 0% improvement. The mean subjective improvement at 2-year follow up was 48.1% [22].

7.4. Aural fullness

Garduno-Anaya et al. pointed out a 48% subjective improvement in aural fullness with ITD [21]. In Ren et al.'s study, aural fullness was complained in 24 of 43 patients. It was disappeared in 4 of 24 patients (16.7%), alleviated in 11 patients (45.8%), and even intensive in 9 patients (37.5%) after ITD injection [12].

Another study included 20 patients with MD; aural fullness was completely resolved in 3 patients (15%) and showed some improvement in 13 patients (65%) after ITD application from ventilation tube by the end of 6 months [19]. In other study including 42 patients treated with ITM, 95.2% had aural fullness before ITM and 65% after ITM by the end of 1-year period [3].

7.5. Live functional activity/quality of life

She et al. found improvement in 94% at 6 months and 87% at 24 months on functional activity after ITM perfusion [4].

In Garduño-Anaya et al.'s study, the initial mean "Dizziness Handicap Inventory" score was 68.7. After receiving ITD, the score was 8.3 at 2 years of follow-up [22].

In Kyrodimos et al.'s study, 30 patients (20 women and 10 men, aged 28–85 years) with MD underwent intratympanic 24 mg/ml of dexamethasone perfusion, and were assessed with the assistance of the Glasgow Benefit Inventory (GBI) questionnaire. Follow-up ranged from 12 to 48 months (mean 30 months) with regard to the GBI responses, nine patients (50%) expressed an overall benefit, while six (33%) expressed no benefit and three patients (17%) complained of negative effect after the intervention [25].

Albu et al. investigated 30 patients with intractable unilateral MD. Before therapy, Dizziness Handicap Inventory (DHI) was 53.2 ± 13.4 and after 12 months follow-up, it was 40.7 ± 16.5. Tinnitus Handicap Inventory (THI) was 28.6 ± 14.3 before therapy and 23.5 ± 12.4 after therapy. Both DHI and THI scores were statistically significant with pre- and posttreatment comparison ($P < 0.001$). At 12 months follow-up, level 1 of Functional Level Score (FLS) was attained in 14 (46.7%) patients and level 2 in 9 (30%) patients [14].

8. Comparison with other treatment methods

Although the exact treatment for MD is still not discovered, several treatment options are available. Caffeine, alcohol, theine and salt (CATS) restriction, diuretics, vasodilators, betahistine, intratympanic injection of gentamicin or corticosteroids, and surgery are most accepted treatment strategies [26].

The initial treatment for MD is diet restriction and oral/parenteral medications. Resistance to this therapy, minimal invasive procedures like intratympanic injections are attempted. The last chance to control symptoms is surgery despite complications (**Figure 1**) [13]. In this section, we compare ITS with other treatment options.

First of all, it must be searched whether ITS has a placebo effect or not. Hu et al. disputed the importance of placebo treatment in MD patients [27]. A double-blind randomized crossover trial using ITD (8 mg/ml) showed no benefit over placebo [28].

Hirvonen et al. also used intratympanic and systemic dexamethasone in 17 patients with MD. They claimed that symptoms of aural fullness, hearing loss, tinnitus, and vertigo did not improve significantly and the clinical use of dexamethasone in MD needs further investigation [16].

On the contrary, another randomized placebo controlled trial showed complete control of vertigo attacks in 82% of patients treated with ITD compared with 57% of those receiving placebo [22].

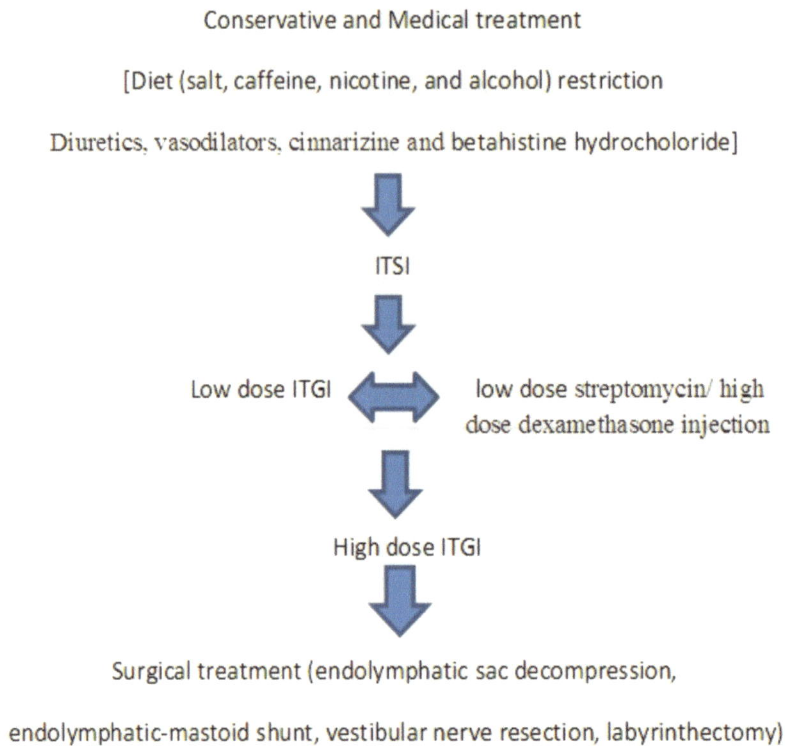

Figure 1. The initial treatment for MD.

Several studies also compare the efficacy of conventional medical treatment and ITS. In Paragache et al.'s study, study group was constituted from 20 patients who was applied ITS and control group was also constituted from 20 patients. Control group patients' diet was free from salt, caffeine, nicotine, and alcohol. Medical management was formed from cinnarizine 25 mg tablets TDS for acute episodes and betahistine hydrochloride 16 mg tablets TDS for continuous treatment. All patients were followed up for 6 months, and results were assessed at 1st, 2nd, 3rd, and 6th months. Vertigo control was 85% at study group and 80% at control group. Hearing loss recovered in three (15%) patients in study group and two (10%) patients in control group. An improvement on SDS was obtained in three (15%) patients in study group and two (10%) patients in control group. Other patients' SDS values were the same. Tinnitus disappeared in two patients in study group and three patients in control group. Tinnitus severity decreased in 12 patients in study group and 10 patients in control group. Aural fullness disappeared in three patients in study group and five patients in control group. Aural fullness severity decreased in 13 patients in study group and 11 patients in control group. They found that both modalities of therapy have almost equal efficacy on MD symptoms, and ITS therapy has an edge over conventional therapy in cases with severe attacks and shorter duration of symptoms [19].

Albu et al. compared the efficacy of ITD and high-dosage betahistine 144 mg/day (48 mg tid). Sixty-six patients with definite unilateral MD were randomly divided in two groups, each comprising 33 patients: Group A received a combination of ITD and identical appearing placebo pills, while Group B received a combination of high-dosage betahistine and IT saline. Fifty-nine patients completed the study and were available at 12 months for analysis, while seven patients (three in Group A and four in Group B) were excluded because of insufficient compliance. The mean number of vertigo attacks per month was recorded at baseline, at 1, 3, and then every 3 months for up to 1 year. Vertigo control was complete (class A) in 14 (46.6%) patients, partial (class B) in 7 (21.2%) patients, and limited (class C or D) in 8 (24.2%) patients in Group A. Vertigo couldn't be controlled in one (3%) patient (class E) in Group A. Vertigo control was complete (class A) in 12 (36.4%) patients, partial (class B) in 5 (15.2%) patients, and limited (class C or D) in 10 (30.4%) patients in Group B. Vertigo couldn't be controlled in two (6.1%) patients (class E) in Group B. Patients whose vertigo attacks couldn't be controlled in both groups were scheduled for ITG therapy. Vertigo control rate wasn't statistically different between two groups. But vertigo attack frequency was 8.6 in Group A and 7.9 in Group B before treatment. It was 1.8 in Group A and 4.3 in Group B after 1 month of treatment. It became 1.5 for Group A and 2.4 for Group B after 3 months of therapy.

According to those results while ITD has a rapid effect to prevent vertigo attack, betahistine and ITD have similar effect on vertigo attack at the end of 3rd month. [14]. Regarding quality of life, while FLS was found level 1 in 14 patients and level 2 in 9 patients in group A, it was found level 1 in 10 patients and level 2 in 9 patients in group B. There was no statistical significance about FLS for both groups [14]. The mean PTA was 57.4 ± 14.7 dB in Group A and 58.2 ± 13.9 dB in Group B before treatment. It became 55.8 ± 15.5 dB for Group A and 56.1 ± 12.5 dB for Group B after 1-year treatment. There was no statistical significance on hearing level and SDS for both groups. A significant reduction in tinnitus assessed by THI at the end of the follow-up was reported in both treatment groups. The difference among the two groups was not significant [14]. They demonstrated that ITD has an immediate effect while higher dosage of betahistine (144 mg/day) is able to get the same outcome only after 3 months of treatment [14].

Intratympanic gentamicin is a traditional treatment for resistant MD. Despite effective vertigo attack control, ototoxicity is a feared complication. Low-dose ITG protocol was used to overcome this complication in some studies [29–31].

Casani et al. compared the effectiveness of ITG and ITD in a study. In this study, patients were randomized and divided into two groups: 32 patients were treated with ITG and 28 patients were treated with ITD. All measurements were obtained immediately before the treatment and were repeated after 1 month, 1 year, and 2 years following the procedure. Vertigo control was complete (class A) in 26 (81.3%) patients, partial (class B) in four (12.5%) patients, and limited (class D) in one (3.2%) patient in ITG group. Vertigo control couldn't be obtained in one patient and vestibular neurectomy was recommended. Vertigo control was complete (class A) in 12 (42.9%) patients, partial (class B) in 5 (17.9%) patients, limited (class C or D) in 9 (32.1%) patients in ITD group. Vertigo control couldn't be obtained in two patients and they were scheduled for gentamicin treatment. There was no statistical significance for vertigo control in both groups ($P < 0.001$) [18]. Level 1 FLS was obtained in 13 (40.6%) patients in ITG group and 11 (39.3%) patients in ITD group at 1-year follow-up. But level 1 FLS was obtained in 22 (71%) patients in ITG group and in 12 (46.1%) patients in ITD group at 2-year follow-up. Although there was no statistical significance at 1-year follow-up, significance was found at 2-year follow-up ($P < 0.05$) [18]. The mean PTA was 58.7 ± 13.3 dB in ITG group and 56.5 ± 13.4 dB in ITD group before treatment. It was 61.3 ± 14.6 and 53.7 ± 15.6 dB in ITG and ITD groups, respectively, after 1 month treatment. At first year, it became 62.3 ± 15.3 and 54.6 ± 16 dB, at second year 64.5 ± 15.5 and 56 ± 17.3 dB for both groups, respectively. There was statistical significance on PTA for both groups ($P > 0.05$) [18]. SDS was found to be 67 ± 19 before treatment, 63.1 ± 20 after 1 month treatment, 61.1 ± 21.1 after 1 year treatment, and 60.3 ± 22.6 after 2 year treatment for ITG group. It was found to be 66.6 ± 16.4 before treatment, 67.5 ± 17.7 after 1 month treatment, 67.1 ± 17.6 after 1 year treatment, and 65.0 ± 18.7 after 2 year treatment for ITD group. The only one value for SDS that reached statistical significance was the difference between pretreatment and after 1 month treatment in ITG group ($P < 0.05$). In the ITD group, no significant variations of SDS were observed during each follow-up ($P > 0.05$) [18]. According to 1995 AAO-HNS criteria, hearing got worse in four (12.9%) patients, not changed in 27 (84.4%) patients, and improved in one (3.1%) patient in ITG group after 2-year treatment. Hearing became worse in 12 (42.9%) patients, not changed in 13 (46.4%) patients, and improved in 3 (10.7%) patients in ITD group after 2-year treatment. Vertigo control was classes A and B in 16 patients in ITD group whose hearing didn't get worse [18]. Total or partial vertigo attack control (class A or B) was over 90% for ITG group and 61% for ITD group after 2-year treatment. According to this study, low-dose ITG therapy was more successful than ITD for vertigo attack control [18]. Regarding the hearing outcome, no statistically significant differences were verified between the two groups in terms of mean PTA and SDS values. On the whole, the mean PTA and SDS values were slightly better for the patients treated with ITD [18]. The authors claimed that low-dose ITG was safe for hearing and efficient for vertigo attack on resistant MD cases [18].

Gabra et al. compared ITM and ITG treatments. There were 89 patients with MD, 47 of them treated with ITG and 42 of them treated with ITM. Two groups were compared for vertigo attack, tinnitus, aural fullness, PTA, and SDS at 0–6 months and 6–12 months. Both groups had similar vertigo attack number before treatment (P: 0.883). Complete vertigo control was obtained in 82.9% in ITG group and 48.1% in ITM group after 6–12 months of treatment (P: 0.004). Tinnitus and aural fullness control were higher in ITG group than in ITM group (P: 0.002). PTA and SDS values were better in ITM group at pretreatment period ($P < 0.001$). But those values became worse in ITM group at 6–12-month control, and difference disappeared between groups ($P > 0.05$) [3]. According to that study, ITG was more effective than ITM to control MD symptoms [3].

Shea et al. suggested a combination of streptomycin and dexamethasone perfusion for MD. The hearing changes and quality-of-life outcomes of 393 cases of streptomycin/dexamethasone inner ear perfusion were searched retrospectively. All patients underwent one or more 3-day treatments consisting of daily intratympanic injections of a low-dose streptomycin (10 mg/ml)/high-dose dexamethasone (24 mg/ml) mixture plus 16 mg of intravenous dexamethasone. The end point for treatment was adequate control of vertigo. The mean PTA change was 0.89 ± 11 dB and the mean SDS change was 0.49 ± 17 after 3-day treatment. Significant hearing loss was detected in 62 (15.7%) patients and hearing loss was severe in 20 (5%) of those patients. Ninety percent of the patients had improved quality of life after treatment and 88% of the patients showed improvement in their "vertigo subscore," a domain within the survey that focuses on vertigo control. According to their results, streptomycin/dexamethasone inner ear perfusion is as safe as other aminoglycoside regimens in the hearing of patients with MD and provides good control of vertigo and a significant improvement in quality of life [32].

Sennaroglu et al. compared three methods to control MD symptoms: ITD, ITG, and decompression of the endolymphatic sac (ESD). Dexamethasone was applied to 24 patients and gentamicin was applied to 16 patients by the ventilation tube way. Surgery of ESD was performed in 25 patients. Vertigo control rates of ITD, ITG, and ESD were 72, 75, and 52%, respectively. Total hearing lost was detected in two patients in ITG group. Hearing level decreased in 9 (38%) patients, improved in 4 (16%) patients, and didn't change in 11 (46%) patients in ITD group. They suggested ITD for patients with the vertiginous symptoms still persisting after 6 months of medical treatment. If patients are resistant to this intervention, ITG could be planned for patients with profound sensorineural hearing loss and ESD could be recommended for patients with normal hearing. Vestibular nerve section could be planned as a last chance to control vertigo attacks for patients with good hearing and labyrinthectomy for patients with profound sensorineural hearing loss [33].

Vestibular nervectomy could be planned as a last chance to control vertigo attacks for good hearing.

Quaranta et al. investigated 38 patients with intractable MD with a minimum of 7 years of follow-up. Twenty patients were treated with endolymphatic-mastoid shunt (EMS) surgery and the remaining eighteen patients refused surgery (natural history, NH group). At the last control, 85% of the patients in EMS group and 74% of the NH patients had complete or substantial control of vertigo. The difference between the two groups was not significant. However, it was significant at 2 and 4 years of follow-up. At 2 years, 65% of the EMS patients had complete or substantial control of vertigo and at 4–6 years in 85% of the cases. Only 32% of the NH patients had complete or substantial control of vertigo at 2 years. This percentage had increased to 50% in the fourth year and to 74% in the sixth year. Hearing results in the two groups were not significantly different. Tinnitus disappeared or decreased in 56% of the EMS patients and in 18% of the NH patients. Sixty-seven percent of the EMS patients and twenty-nine percent of the NH patients reported that their aural fullness disappeared. Consequently, vertigo attack reduction was observed earlier in EMS patients than in those who refused surgery [34].

9. Conclusions

Although the fact that definitive treatment of MD has not been found yet, several treatment options are used to control the MD symptoms. Different success rates of symptom relief are given in literature for each option. However, common agreed decision is that ITS can be used in patients with intractable MD to conservative and medical treatment before intratympanic gentamicin and surgical treatments.

Author details

Fatih Oghan[1]*, Ibrahim Erdim[2], Metin Çeliker[3], Muhammet Fatih Topuz[4], Ahmet Uluat[4], Onur Erdogan[4] and Sinan Aksoy[4]

*Address all correspondence to: fatihoghan@hotmail.com

1 Faculty of Medicine, Department of ORL&HNS, Dumlupinar University, Kutahya, Turkey

2 Tokat Erbaa Hospital, Tokat, Turkey

3 Recep Tayyip Erdogan University Research Hospital, Rize, Turkey

4 SB DPU Evliya Celebi Research Hospital, Kutahya, Turkey

References

[1] McCabe BF. Autoimmune sensorineural hearing loss. Annals of Otology & Rhinology. 1979;**88**:585-590

[2] Cheng KC, Mastsvoka H, Lee KM, Kim NS, Krug MS, Kwon SS, et al. Proto-oncogene Raf-1 as an autoantigen in Méniére's disease. Annals of Otology, Rhinology & Layngology. 2000;**109**:1093-1098

[3] Gabra N, Saliba I. The effect of intratympanic methylprednisolone and gentamicin injection on Méniére's Disease. Otolaryngology—Head and Neck Surgery. 2013;**148** (4):642-647

[4] She W, Lv L, Du X, Li H, Dai Y, Lu L, Ma X, Chen F. Long-term effects of intratympanic methylprednisolone perfusion treatment on intractable Ménière's disease. The Journal of Laryngology & Otology. 2015;**129**:232-237

[5] Rarey KE, Curtis LM. Receptors for glucocorticoids in the human inner ear. Otolaryngology—Head and Neck Surgery. 1996;**115**:38-41

[6] Lohuis PJ, Ten Cate WJ, Patterson KE. Modulation of rat stria vascularis in the absence of circulating adrenocorticosteroids. Acta Otolaryngologica (Stockh). 1990;**110**:348-356

[7] Tomiyama S, Nonaka M, Gotoh Y, Ikezono I, Yagi I. Immunological approach to Méniére's disease: Vestibular immune injury following immune reaction of the endolymphatic sac. The Journal of Otorhinology & Laryngology. 1994;**56**:11-18

[8] Merchant SN, Adams JC, Nadol JB Jr. Pathophysiology of Méniére's syndrome: Are symptoms caused by endolymphatic hydrops? Otology & Neurotology. 2005;**26**:74-81

[9] Fukushima M, Kitahara T, Fuse Y, et al. Changes in aquaporin expression in the inner ear of the rat after i.p. injection of steroids. Acta Oto-Laryngologica Supplementum. 2004;**553**:13-18

[10] Shirwany NA, Seidman MD, Tang W. Effects of transtympanic injection of steroids on cochlear blood flow, auditory sensitivity and histology in guinea pigs. American Journal of Otolaryngology. 1998;**19**:230-235

[11] Otake H, Yamamoto H, Teranishi M, Sone M, Nakashima T. Cochlear blood flow during occlusion and reperfusion of the anterior inferior cerebellar artery: Effect of topical application of dexamethasone to the round window. Acta Otolaryngology. 2009;**129**:127-131

[12] Ren H, Yin T, Lu Y, Kong W, Ren J. Intratympanic dexamethasone injections for refractory Méniére's disease. International Journal of Clinical and Experimental Medicine. 2015;**8**(4):6016-6023

[13] Barrs DM, Keyser JS, Stallworth C, McElveen JT. Intratympanic steroid injections for intractable Méniére's disease. Laryngoscope. 2001;**111**:2100-2104

[14] Albu S, Chirtes F, Trombitas V, Nagy A, Marceanu L, Babighian G, Trabalzini F. Intratympanic dexamethasone versus high dosage of betahistine in the treatment of intractable unilateral Méniére disease. American Journal of Otolaryngology. 2015 Mar–Apr;**36**(2):205-209

[15] Parnes LS, Sun AH, Freeman DJ. Corticosteroid pharmacokinetics in the inner ear fluids: An animal study followed by clinical application. Laryngoscope. 1999;**109**:1-17

[16] Hirvonen TP, Peltomaa M, Ylikoski J. Intratympanic and systemic dexamethasone for Méniére's disease. ORL Journal of Otorhinolaryngology and its Related Specialties. 2000;**62**:117-120

[17] She W, Dai Y, Du X, Yu C, Chen F, Wang J et al. Hearing evaluation of intratympanic methylprednisolone perfusion for refractory sudden sensorineural hearing loss. Otolaryngology—Head and Neck Surgery. 2010;**142**:266-271

[18] Casani AP, Piaggi P, Cerchiai N, Seccia V, Franceschini SS, Dallan I. Intratympanic treatment of intractable unilateral Méniére disease: Gentamicin or dexamethasone? A randomized controlled trial. Otolaryngology—Head and Neck Surgery. 2012 Mar;**146**(3):430-437

[19] Paragache G, Panda NK, Ragunathan M, Sridhara. Intratympanic dexamethasone application in Méniére's disease—Is it superior to conventional therapy? Indian Journal of Otolaryngology—Head and Neck Surgery. 2005 Jan;**57**(1):21-23

[20] Hamid MA. Intratympanic dexamethasone perfusion in Méniére's. In: Presented at the Spring Meeting of the American Neurotology Society; Palm Desert, CA; May 2001. p. 12

[21] Boleas-Aguirre MS, Lin FR, Della Santina CC, Minor LB, Carey JP. Longitudinal results with intratympanic dexamethasone in the treatment of Ménière's disease. Otology & Neurotology. 2008;**29**(1):33-38

[22] Garduño-Anaya MA, Couthino De Toledo H, Hinojosa-González R, Pane-Pianese C, Ríos-Castañeda LC. Dexamethasone inner ear perfusion by intratympanic injection in unilateral Ménière's disease: A two-year prospective, placebo-controlled, double-blind, randomized trial. Otolaryngology—Head and Neck Surgery. 2005 Aug;**133**(2):285-294

[23] Kaplan DM, Hehar SS, Bance ML, Rutka JA. Intentional ablation of vestibular function using commercially available topical gentamicin-betamethasone eardrops in patients with Méniére's disease: Further evidence for topical eardrop ototoxicity. Laryngoscope. 2002 Apr;**112**(4):689-695

[24] Hillman TM, Arriaga MA, Chen DA. Intratympanic steroids: Do they acutely improve hearing in cases of cochlear hydrops? Laryngoscope. 2003;**113**:1903-1907

[25] Kyrodimos E, Aidonis I, Skalimis A, Sismanis A. Use of Glasgow benefit inventory (GBI) in Méniére's disease managed with intratympanic dexamethasone perfusion: Quality of life assessment. Auris Nasus Larynx. 2011 Apr;**38**(2):172-177

[26] Coelho DH, Lalwani AK. Medical management of Méniére's disease. Laryngoscope. 2008;**118**:1099-1108

[27] Hu A, Parnes LS. Intratympanic steroids for inner ear disorders: A review. Audiology and Neurotology. 2009;**14**:373-382

[28] Silverstein H, Isaacson JE, Olds MJ, Rowan PT, Rosenberg S. Dexamethasone inner ear perfusion for the treatment of Méniére's disease: A prospective, randomized, double-blind, crossover trial. American Journal of Otolaryngology. 1998;**19**:196-201

[29] Longridge NS, Mallinson AI. Low-dose intratympanic gentamicin treatment for dizziness in Méniére's disease. Journal of Otolaryngology. 2000;**29**:35-39

[30] Harner SG, Drisco CL, Facer GW, et al. Long-term follow-up of transtympanic gentamicin for Méniére's syndrome. Otology & Neurotology. 2001;**22**:210-214

[31] Quaranta A, Scaringi A, Aloidi A, Quaranta N, Salonna I. Intratympanic therapy for Méniére's disease: Effect of administration of low concentration of gentamicin. Acta Otolaryngology. 2001;**121**:387-392

[32] Shea PF, Richey PA, Wan JY, Stevens SR. Hearing results and quality of life after streptomycin/dexamethasone perfusion for Méniére's disease. Laryngoscope. 2012 Jan;**122**(1):204-211

[33] Sennaroglu L, Sennaroglu G, Gursel B, Dini FM. Intratympanic dexamethasone, intratympanic gentamicin, and endolymphatic sac surgery for intractable vertigo in Méniére's disease. Otolaryngology—Head and Neck Surgery. 2001 Nov;**125**(5):537-543

[34] Quaranta A, Marini F, Sallustio V. Long-term outcome of Méniére's disease: Endolymphatic mastoid shunt versus natural history. Audiology and Neuro-otology. 1998;**3**:54-60